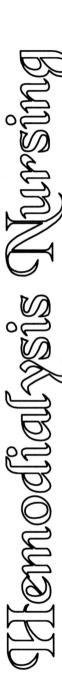

Blood & Chemistry

A Monograph
for Continuing Education

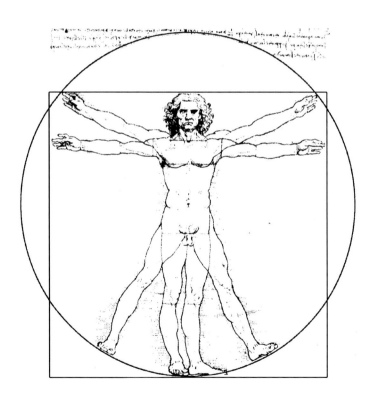

Joanne D. Pittard MS, RN

Blood and Uremia Monograph, First Edition

Author: Joanne D. Pittard MS, RN

Editor: John R De Palma, MD

Publisher: Hemodialysis, Inc

Copyright: This work is the intellectual property of the author and protected by copyright ©. No part may be reproduced or used in any form or by any means –graphic, electronic, or mechanical, including photocopying– without the written permission from the author.

Inside Cover: "The Proportions of the Human Figure, After Vitruvius"

Artist: Leonardo Da Vinci

Date: 1492

Location: Academy Museum, Venice, Italy

Editor's Note:

The graphic on the inside cover identifies this series of monographs. It is redrawn from but not exactly the same (the circle and square do not touch the figure's finger tips) as Leonardo's pen and ink drawing for Vitruvius's book. Leonardo's mirror writing above the figure of a man states: "The navel is naturally placed in the centre of the human body, and if a circle be described of a man lying with his face upward and his hands and feet extended, it will touch his fingers and his toes. It is not alone by a circle that the human body is thus circumscribed, as may be seen by placing it within a square. For if we measure from the feet to the crown of the head, and then across the arms fully extended, we should find the latter measure equally to the former; so that the lines at right angles to each other enclosing the figure, and form a square."

Cover Graphic: Scanning electron microscope, photo of erythrocytes

Provider Information

The Author

The author of this monograph is Joanne D. Pittard MS, RN. The material and graphics are a super-set of Joanne's training manual 𝕳𝖊𝖒𝖔𝖉𝖎𝖆𝖑𝖞𝖘𝖎𝖘 𝕹𝖚𝖗𝖘𝖎𝖓𝖌, Sixth Edition, Version 6.8. That training manual was first published in 1987 as lecture topics and course objectives for the one semester college nursing course "Hemodialysis Nursing." The manual is now a six-hundred and seventy-four (674) page graphic and text *outline* of her training program. Joanne has taught that course at Glendale Community College, Glendale, California since 1975. In 1984, California legislation used her nursing course as the model for training and education for Patient Care Technician (PCT) education and certification. The course now attracts Registered Nurses (RNs) from several Western states. It is the oldest college level RN program of didactic and *practicum* dialysis teaching in the United States.

About 1992, at specific request from the publisher, her manual was made available to educators by mail. The response was remarkable. That response, and the letters asking for more detailed information about dialytic nursing care led to Joanne's first monograph, "Principles of Dialysis," printed in March 1998. Advertising consisted of one direct mailing to RNs in November 1998. Orders for her monograph continue as RNs and PCTs refer their friends. The original monograph has been updated and renamed to "Principles of Dialysis 2000." It is over thirty (30) pages longer than the original monograph.

Joanne's academic association is:

Joanne Duffney Pittard MS, RN
Professor of Allied Health
Glendale Community College, Glendale, CA

A Monograph as a Teaching Instrument

A monograph is a writing, either in essay or book length, on a single or specific subject. This monograph comprises some, not all, of the elements needed to understand the interrelationships between the patient's blood and the dialysis treatment.

Many of the graphics and material in this writing are especially drawn and written for it. The material is derived from Joanne's hands on educational experience and her role as a nursing consultant and advisor to the ESRD industry. We think and believe that this publication is unique. Joanne was a dialysis nursing supervisor, is a hands on educator, and she presently serves as a nursing and education expert in the dialysis industry.

The Publisher

Purchasing copies of this monograph, certification of educational credits, and inquiries relating to this monograph are handled by the publisher:

HEMODIALYSIS, INC.
710 West Wilson Avenue
Glendale, CA 91203-2409
Tel: 818 500-8736
http://www.**Hemodialysis-Inc.com**

Provider Information

Hemodialysis, Inc. (**Hi**) is the provider for this monograph. **Hi** is a licensed health-care corporation based in Southern California. **Hi** is provider approved by the California Board of Registered Nursing, Provider Number CEP2359. Part of **Hi**'s mission and goals is to foster quality dialysis care for ESRD patients and to provide quality education for ESRD personnel. Continuing education credits in the form of thirty (30) contact hours for this monograph will be given.

To Earn thirty (30) Contact Hours of Continuing Education:

1   Read the introduction, objectives, and entire monograph.

2   Take the attached test and fill in all answers.

3   Fill in the registration information on the answer form.

4   Mail the **original** registration and answer form to the publisher within one (1) year of purchase of the monograph.

5   **Do not fax or mail a copy of the registration and answer form.** We must have the original form to process your test and complete your registration.

Mail Test & Registration To:

HEMODIALYSIS, INC.
710 West Wilson Ave
Glendale, CA 91203-2409

Office hours – Monday through Friday – 8:30 AM to 5:00 PM

Certification for Regular Orders

You will be notified of your test results within four (4) weeks after receipt of the registration and answer form. We urge you to send the answer form by registered or certified mail. We are unable to verify receipt by regular mail. If you pass, a certificate for earned contact hours will be awarded by Hemodialysis, Inc. If you fail the test, you may submit another answer form within thirty (30) days with no surcharges.

Special Handling of Orders in USA

A surcharge of fifty USA dollars ($50.00) is added to the monograph price for orders with:

1 Turn around time of less than four (4) weeks

2 Any requests not covered in the preceding paragraph, titled: "Certification for Regular Orders."

FedEx Mailing in USA

A surcharge of fifty USA dollars ($50.00) is added for any order requiring FedEx type mailing as part of Special Handling. Maximum surcharge of Special Handling is a total of $50.00.

Books mailed First Class

We ship all books by first class mail –with delivery confirmation– inside the USA.

Mailing outside the USA

All mailings outside the USA will require the purchaser to forward an additional sum for mailing and handling.

The Editor

John R De Palma, MD, FACP is the editor of this monograph. All data come from respected medical research, analysis of patient data, and the application of standard statistical analysis. Pre-prints of this monograph were submitted to authorities in: internal medicine, hematology, nephrology, hemodialysis machinery, and nursing. Thus, this one writing represents a unique, multi-disciplinary collection of data and knowledge. The editor would be greatly pleased to receive any written comments at Hemodialysis, Inc.

The monograph is lightly referenced and heavily researched. Much of its content is contained in well-known medical textbooks and was taught in post-graduate medicine and nephrology, *see* Books of Authority on page 175.

Any praise for: topics included, graphics, clarity of thought, general content, objectives, nursing care plans and nursing intelligence displayed in this monograph should be addressed to Professor Pittard at Hemodialysis, Inc. Professor Pittard provides both the inspiration and the content of this monograph.

Desktop Publishing

All desktop computer work (text and graphic) is done using a variety of simple Windows™ 98 personal computers (PCs). Vector (line and formula based) graphics are drawn by Joanne using Microsoft's Power Point 7.0a. Raster (bitmap) graphics are either drawn or edited from digitized photographs using Adobe's PhotoShop 3.0.4. Examples of these digitized graphics include an edited photograph of Joanne's left arm for the graphic, Loading Dose of Heparin on page 102, and Doctor De Palma's fountain pen on page 117.

Electronic Hypertext Version of the Monograph

Microsoft's Excel 5.0c and 7.0a is used for all statistical analysis and graphs. Microsoft Word 7.0a is used to prepare the twenty-four (24) files. Adobe's FrameMaker 5.5.6 is used to collate the files and prepare the monograph both for publication and to generate the full-color electronic Adobe Reader document which mirrors this monograph. That full-color electronic file is available as a separate reference, teaching, and resource tool.

Author's Preface

This publication is written for health-care personnel who provide professional help to patients with End Stage Renal Disease (ESRD). The information in this monograph is important and essential for: registered nurses (RNs), licensed vocational nurses (LVNs), hemodialysis patient care technicians (PCTs), machine technicians, and physicians; everyone who provides direct ESRD patient care. Administrative and health-care personnel who are not involved in the day-to-day and routine care of ESRD patients by dialysis machinery will find a compilation of vital material which impacts on quality of care that is unavailable in any other single source.

The mission and goal of this monograph is to improve the delivery of care for ESRD patients. RNs have the benefit of nursing school. PCTs have not had the advantage of this formal introduction and education for care of the sick. We have purposely included fundamental information, in order to educate the many PCTs that have not had the advantage of nursing school. PCTs now care for the majority of dialysis patients in the United States of America (USA).

One of the conundrums in teaching is to know what information to cover and what to omit. What facts are vital for the nurse or PCT to know? What information is non-essential but interesting? My intent is to focus on the key points and relevant correlations of anatomy and physiology and the hemodialysis process. We hope that this monograph will help the reader to deliver a safer dialysis treatment and to improve the patient's quality of life.

Features of this monograph include:

1   contact hours for continuing education credits, thirty (30)
2   diagrams
3   ESRD formulas not found in any other single text or reference
4   examination questions and test
5   glossary of ESRD terms

6 hyper-linked electronic file in full color which mirrors the content of this monograph; available as a separate educational device to augment this monograph

7 monograph objectives

8 new concepts in nursing and medical care for ESRD patients

9 primer on SI units and conversion tables for SI units

10 raster graphics from digitized photographs

11 table of contents and index

12 tables of values

13 vector graphics from Microsoft PowerPoint 7.0a.

I am grateful to all of my past students who helped to keep me on track over the years. I am indebted to John R De Palma, MD, my mentor and editor.

Joanne D Pittard

Joanne D Pittard MS, RN

Table of Contents

Table of Contents

Table of Contents

Post Test

Index

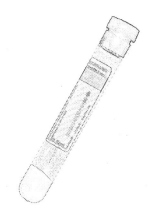

Introduction

This monograph, "Blood and Uremia" discusses the composition and function of blood and how careful handing of the patient's blood relates to the treatment of patients on hemodialysis.

Basic and advanced knowledge of the composition and function of whole blood is important for all ESRD healthcare personnel.

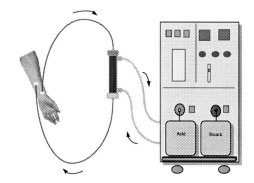

Figure 1 - Hemodialysis system

Acute and chronic hemodialysis therapy underpins all real and artificial organ medicine and surgical procedures. Acute hemodialysis is often needed post organ transplantation.

About one out of every one-thousand (1/1000) citizens of the United States of America (Americans) are treated by chronic hemodialysis. Most Americans either have a family member or know someone being treated by hemodialysis.

We hope this monograph will help the reader to apply new knowledge to the entire hemodialysis process and better understand: blood, the anemia of uremia, and anticoagulation therapy.

Topics:

1 role of erythropoietin in red blood cell production
2 causes of anemia
3 assessment of anemia
4 historical perspective of anemia in renal failure

5   the current treatment approaches to correct the state of anemia

6   anticoagulation therapy

7   implementation of appropriate nursing intervention for the ESRD patient

8   the interrelationship of vitamins, nutrition, and anemia

9   the concepts concerning adequacy of dialysis care as it relates to treatment of anemia

10 basic histology and physiology of blood

11 issues that impact on the ability to deliver care.

Objectives

1 List a minimum of six different functions of blood.

2 Identify five characteristics of blood.

3 Describe the composition of blood.

4 Identify the three types of cells in blood and briefly describe their function.

5 Describe the constituents of plasma water.

6 State the normal value for total plasma proteins.

7 Describe briefly how plasma proteins maintain the osmolarity of the intravascular compartment.

8 Differentiate between plasma and serum.

9 Identify the four main blood groups or blood types.

10 Identify the hormone responsible for erythropoiesis.

11 Describe briefly, the process of erythropoiesis.

12 Identify three dietary factors that influence red blood cell production.

13 List two blood tests that indicate a patient's state of nutrition and give the acceptable range for each.

14 Describe the significance of iron and erythropoiesis.

15 Define the word hematocrit.

16 Identify the normal range of the hematocrit for the general population without renal failure, differentiate between males and females.

17 Differentiate between a spun hematocrit and a laboratory hematocrit.

18 Define the word hemoglobin.

19 Identify the usual range for hemoglobin.

20 Identify the overall function of the white blood cell (WBC).

21 List the different types of white blood cells and briefly describe their individual function; include the usual percent seen in a differential count.

22   Identify the primary reason to perform a white blood cell count on a dialysis patient.

23   Identify three causes of an elevated white blood cell count.

24   Explain the appropriate time to collect a blood specimen for an accurate WBC count.

25   Identify what a complete blood count (CBC) measures.

26   Describe the function of platelets.

27   Briefly describe the blood coagulation system.

28   Describe the role of platelets and clotting factors in the normal clotting process.

29   Describe the substance fibrin.

30   Define the word hemostasis.

31   Identify three factors that affect hemostasis.

32   Explain the significance of the dialyzing fluid having a similar osmolarity as plasma.

33   Identify the need for implementing standard precautions in the dialysis setting.

34   Identify three blood-borne pathogens.

35   List five precautions to use; to prevent the transmission of blood-borne pathogens from patient to patient and to protect the health-care worker.

36   Define the term anemia.

37   Identify three causes of red blood cell (RBC) deficiency in the ESRD patient.

38   List three tools to assess anemia in the ESRD patient.

39   List six signs and/or symptoms of anemia.

40   Differentiate between a Hgb and Hct as an assessment tool for uremic anemia.

41   State the primary reason for reduced erythropoiesis in the ESRD patient.

42   Identify six causes of anemia in the ESRD patient, in addition to reduced erythropoiesis.

43   Describe the significance of the reticulocyte count.

44   Describe the condition methemoglobinemia.

45   Define the word hemolysis.

46   Identify four potential causes of hemolysis.

47   List four signs and or symptoms of hemolysis that a patient would experience.

48   Describe how to assess for hemolysis.

49   Describe the appropriate nursing management and/or intervention when hemolysis occurs.

50   List four ways to prevent hemolysis from occurring.

51   Describe the relationship of iron deficiency and anemia.

52   Identify the two blood tests used in iron assessment, state the acceptable laboratory values and state their significance.

53   Identify three different ways that a hemodialysis patient can experience blood loss.

54   List six different approaches in the hemodialysis environment to prevent blood loss in a patient.

55   Describe the most current interventions used to correct iron deficiency in the hemodialysis patient.

56   Describe a few problems with the use of oral iron preparations.

57   Identify the intravenous medication that is currently the most popular method of correcting iron deficiency.

58   Identify potential problems with the infusion of intravenous iron dextran preparations.

59   Identify the best way to prevent anaphylaxis and/or an allergic response when giving intravenous iron.

60   List six signs and/or symptoms of an anaphylactic reaction and/or an allergic response.

61   Discuss the nursing intervention in the treatment of anaphylaxis.

62   Identify the newly approved intravenous iron supplement.

63   Describe the relationship of anemia with the following: 1) folic acid deficiency, 2) osteitis fibrosa cystica, 3) aluminum toxicity, and 4) blood transfusions.

64   List five treatment approaches to correct anemia.

65   Describe briefly, the source for the drug known as recombinant human erythropoietin (epoetin alfa) and its commercial production.

66   Discuss the indications and usage of epoetin in the ESRD patient.

67   Describe the usual dose and method of administration of epoetin.

68   Identify the target hematocrit range for patient's on epoetin.

69   Identify the major cause of delayed or diminished response to epoetin therapy.

70   Identify the recommended tests and desired blood levels for assessing the patient's iron stores to assure adequate erythropoiesis.

71   Identify three parameters to be monitored in addition to iron stores for patients on epoetin therapy.

72   Identify any toxic or allergic effects have been observed with patients on epoetin therapy.

73   Identify four possible impacts of epoetin therapy on the dialysis prescription and/or procedure.

74   State the formula for calculating a mean blood pressure.

75   Calculate a mean blood pressure (MAP) from a blood pressure of 120/80.

76   Identify nursing interventions that can be utilized during the dialysis treatment to maintain the patient's hematocrit and prevent further anemia.

77   Define the word anticoagulation.

78   Explain the need for anticoagulation therapy during dialysis.

79   Describe the indications and usage for heparin sodium in the hemodialysis setting.

80   Identify two exogenous sources of heparin.

81   State the chemical composition of heparin and give its molecular weight.

82   State how heparin sodium works, list a minimum of four points.

83   Identify the concentration of the heparin sodium solution used during dialysis.

84   Identify five variables to consider when determining heparin requirements.

85   Identify the heparin dose for hemodialysis, adjusted for no residual renal function.

86   Explain the significance of the plasma half-life of heparin.

87   List five conditions that may retard the activity of heparin, necessitating larger doses.

88   List five conditions that may prolong the activity of heparin, necessitating smaller doses.

89   Identify the appropriate route of administration of heparin during dialysis and how soon it takes effect.

90   State the usual and customary dosage used for heparin sodium for the initial dose and hourly sustaining dose for patients.

91   List three methods used to administer heparin therapy for hemodialysis.

92   Describe when and how the "loading dose" is given.

93   Describe when and how the continuous or sustaining dose is given.

94   Identify a problem with intermittent heparin therapy.

95   Identify a minimum of five complications of too much or an overdose of heparin therapy.

96   Identify a minimum of five complications of administering an inadequate amount of heparin.

97   List five methods to avoid blood clotting of the extracorporeal circuit during hemodialysis.

98   Identify a minimum of six nursing interventions to assure proper heparinization of the patient and extracorporeal circuit.

99   Explain the significance of the Clinical Laboratory Improvement Amendment (CLIA) and its impact in caring for the ESRD patient.

100   List five advantages of using the ACT method to monitor anticoagulation therapy.

101   Explain the significance of monitoring the use of oral anticoagulants in the hemodialysis patient.

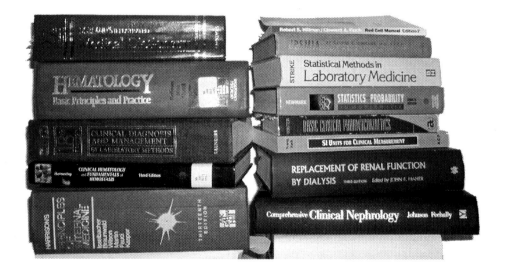

Blood

Blood is a complex liquid which performs special and vital functions. Blood is an organ. The study of blood is known as hematology. Blood is contained in and carried by blood vessels. The heart's major function is to pump blood through the body's network of blood vessels to all living cells. In health, blood is confined to the intravascular compartment, ie: within blood vessels.

Functions of Blood

Blood transports oxygen (O_2) transferred from lung capillaries to all body tissues. Carbon dioxide (CO_2), the gaseous product of metabolism, is transferred to blood at the cell level and transported to the lungs for elimination.

Foods are digested, transformed by the liver, and delivered as fats, sugars, and amino acids to cells by the blood. Cellular wastes are transported by the blood to the kidneys, lungs, and liver for excretion or detoxification.

Special organs or cells produce secretions, hormones, and enzymes, which the blood transports to various tissues. One hormone, erythropoietin, is produced primarily by the kidneys. Blood transports erythropoietin to the bone marrow to aid in the production of red blood cells (RBCs).

Blood aids in the regulation of body temperature by distributing heat produced in active muscles. Acid-base buffers in the blood, help to maintain the body's acid base balance.

The white blood cells (WBCs) and special globulins in the blood are the first line of defense in protecting the body from outside invaders such as:

1   viruses
2   bacteria
3   foreign proteins and antigens.

Characteristics of Blood

The color of blood, is determined by the color of its RBCs. When the RBCs are rich in oxygen, the blood is bright red. This blood is commonly referred to as arterial blood. As the hemoglobin releases oxygen to the cells, the RBCs darken, becoming more red-blue. This is commonly called venous blood.

Approximately seventy-five percent (75%) of blood is in the venous system, five percent (5%) in the capillaries and the remaining twenty percent (20%) is in the arterial system.

Approximately seven percent (7%) of the normal body's weight is blood. A person weighing 70 kilograms (Kg) has approximately 4.9Kg or 4,900 milliliters (mL) of blood. The cellular elements, proteins, and other substances make blood about five (5) times more viscous than water.

Composition of Blood

Blood is made up of several types of cells, electrolytes, compounds, and fats suspended in a clear straw-colored liquid called plasma. Plasma is the major body-fluid in the intravascular compartment, (Figure 2).

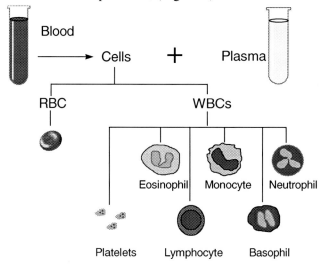

Figure 2 - Components of Blood

There are three (3) different types of cells in blood:

1   RBCs

2   WBCs

3   platelets.

Spinning whole blood in a centrifuge at high centrifugal force separates the blood cells from the liquid portion of the blood.

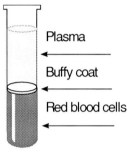

Plasma

Buffy coat

Red blood cells

Figure 3 - Centrifuged Blood

Centrifugation layers the blood components. The heaviest layer at the bottom of the test tube, with increasingly lighter substances layering above.

The RBCs layer at the bottom of the test tube. The WBCs are next (buffy coat) and platelets may form a thin line above the WBCs, (Figure 3).

If the blood is drawn from a patient who has not eaten, "fasting state specimen," the top layer is clear plasma. If the person has eaten, then lipids absorbed from the GI tract will render the plasma cloudy or milky in appearance.

Some dialysis patients continue to have lipids circulating in their plasma long after they have eaten. These dialysis patients may have cloudy plasma even in a fasting state. Their blood may look like "strawberries and cream" when drawn.

This persistent hyperlipidemia, usually due to elevated triglycerides, is associated with accelerated vascular disease in these patients. If a patient's fasting blood sample contains cloudy plasma, the patient's physician should be so advised. Additional tests to pin point the type of lipid abnormality may be indicated.

Cells account for about forty five (45%) percent of blood. The plasma portion of the blood makes up the remaining fifty-five percent (55%).

Note: If the plasma is yellow, "jaundiced," rather than straw colored, it may indicate gall bladder or liver disease. An elevation in the serum bilirubin is the common cause of yellow plasma. In dialysis patients, this may be an early finding of viral hepatitis.

Composition of Plasma

Ninety two percent (92%) of plasma is water and the remaining eight percent (8%) solutes. Most of the plasma solutes, seven (7) of the eight percent (8%), are proteins. The remaining one percent (1%) include:

1 *nutrients;* carbohydrates, amino acids, and lipids

2 *inorganic salts;* (electrolytes) such as calcium, magnesium, sodium, potassium, chlorides, sulfates, phosphates, and carbonates

3 *vitamins*

4 *hormones*

5 *enzymes*

6 *gases;* oxygen, carbon dioxide, and nitrogen

7 *waste products;* urea, uric acid, creatinine, and lactic acid.

Plasma Proteins

The main plasma proteins are:

1 albumin

2 globulin

3 fibrinogen.

The normal value for total plasma proteins in the blood is six to eight grams per deciliter (6 - 8 g/dL). Plasma proteins aid in the return of ultrafiltered fluid through the use of osmotic pressure. Blood enters the capillaries under pressure from the arterioles, (Figure 4). Ultrafiltration occurs and plasma water crosses the capillary membrane to the surrounding tissues. The plasma proteins present in blood plasma

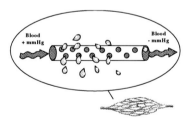

Figure 4 - Capillary Ultrafiltration

are too large to cross the openings in the capillary membrane. They remain inside the capillaries. They create an osmotic force that returns the extracellular fluid (ECF) back into the blood compartment at the venous end of the capillaries.

Osmosis is the movement of water across a semipermeable membrane from an area of lower solute concentration to an area of higher solute concentration. The plasma proteins and the physical process of osmosis prevent a progressive loss of ECF into the interstitial space, (Figure 5).

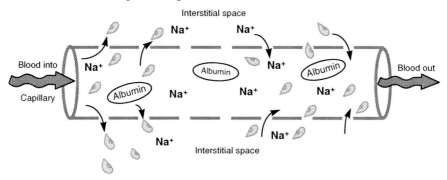

Figure 5 - Capillary Return of ECF

Albumin, normally accounts for about fifty-five percent (55%) of all the plasma proteins. The serum albumin level is commonly used to evaluate the nutritional status of the patient as it is felt to reflect the protein stores in the body.

Fibrinogen and prothrombin are normally inactive substances present in the plasma. They both play an important role in the blood clotting process.

Globulins function as key components in the immune system. Synthesis of plasma proteins occurs in the liver cells.

Blood Cell Production

The different types of blood cells originate from a single stem cell; an ancestor cell. The maturation of the different blood cell types is similar to the development of a family tree. The stem cell divides into two main lines or lineage's; the myeloid stem cell and lymphoid stem cell.

Different hormones cause a specific type of blood cell to develop and mature with their own unique function and specialization. These hormones are known as

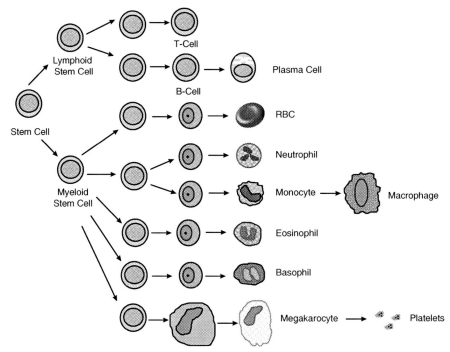

Figure 6 - Maturation of Blood Cells

hemopoietins or hormones that make blood. The stem cells reside in the bone marrow, where the development of individualized cells takes place, (Figure 6).

Red Blood Cells

An erythrocyte is a mature RBC. Erythrocytes are unique living cells. They have no nucleus to allow protein synthesis. Their energy metabolism depends almost exclusively on glucose. They are biconcave, with a thicker rim, average eight microns (8μ) in length and two microns (2μ) in width.

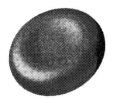

Figure 7 - RBC

The erythrocyte cell membrane is elastic, allowing it to deform and fold to fit through the smaller diameter of the capillaries.

Erythrocytes contain –as their principal protein– hemoglobin (Hgb). Hgb is an iron-protein with a molecular weight of 68,000 daltons. Hgb gives the RBC its red color and comprises thirty-three percent (33%) of its intracellular protein. There is about one milligram (1 mg) of elemental iron in each milliliter of normal RBCs. Four (4) polypeptide chains make up Hgb. When freed from the RBC by intravascular hemolysis, these polypeptide chains break down into molecules about one-half their original size. These smaller molecules are still too large to dialyze to any significant degree. Dialysate does not turn red with intravascular hemolysis; only with actual leakage of RBCs into the dialysate.

The Hgb of the RBC transports oxygen and carbon dioxide (CO_2). Oxygen dissolved in the plasma and in the red blood cell water, moves in and out of the red cell by way of diffusion.

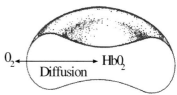

Figure 8 - *Hgb Transport*

The normal hemoglobin level in the blood is twelve to sixteen grams per deciliter (12 - 16 g/dL). Age and sex affect the normal levels of Hgb.

The average normal adult RBC count is five million per cubic millimeter (5,000,000/mm^3). The normal RBC life span is about 120 ± 20 days. Thus the *lower* normal value of RBC survival is 100 days; the *higher* is 140 days. The old and more fragile RBCs are removed from circulation -mainly- by the spleen.

Erythropoiesis

Erythropoiesis means the manufacture of RBCs. Ninety percent (90%) of the hormone erythropoietin, is produced by cells in the kidney. The liver produces most of the remaining ten percent (10%).

Erythropoietin production is in response to oxygen deficiency in the tissues (tissue hypoxia). When special renal cells sense a low tissue partial pressure of oxygen (pO_2), they release erythropoietin. The secreted erythropoietin, now in the blood stream, travels to the red bone marrow.

In the adult, the red bone marrow, which manufactures RBCs, is contained in bones[1] of the:

1   cranium
2   proximal humerus

3 pelvis

4 ribs

5 proximal femur

Erythropoietin acts as a growth hormone on marrow stem cells. In about a week to eight (8) days, after a single hormone stimulus, mature RBCs and some reticulocytes enter the blood stream. It does not require a continuous stimulus of erythropoietin to cause RBCs to be manufactured. This explains the ability of dialysis units to administer recombinant human erythropoietin (epoetin) only on dialysis days and still accomplish erythropoiesis.

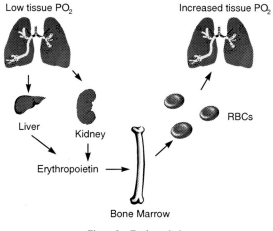

Figure 9 - Erythropoiesis

As RBCs are manufactured and the tissue oxygen concentration increases in the tissues of the kidneys and liver, the release of erythropoietin decreases. The production of erythropoietin is *inversely* related to tissue oxygenation. The release of an increasing number of RBCs into the circulation raises the oxygen carrying capacity of the blood, (Figure 9).

Reticulocytes

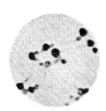

Figure 10 - Reticulocyte

Newly formed RBCs leave the bone marrow as immature cells containing residual ribonucleic acid (RNA) material. They are called reticulocytes, because the RNA stains as strains or a reticulum, (Figure 10). Reticulocytes are somewhat larger and less concave than mature RBCs. Their number and percent is the simplest and most practical measure of RBC production, or how rapidly the bone marrow makes RBCs.

Counting Reticulocytes

Reticulocytes can be seen by preparing a blood smear on a glass slide and then staining *first* with a vital dye such as methylene blue and *second* with Wright's stain. These immature cells may then be counted. They can not be seen on regular Wright stain which is normally used to evaluate RBC size and shape. Reticulocytes normally comprise about one percent (1%) of the total RBC count; and this is consistent with the normal loss of one percent (1%) of RBCs per day. "Reticulocyte Count" beginning on page 48 discusses the formulas for reticulocyte assessment.

Polychromatophilic RBCs

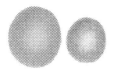

Figure 11 - RBCs

If the reticulocyte count is elevated secondary to increased erythropoietic stimulation, there will be cells on the Wright's stain smear, that are somewhat larger than mature RBCs with a blue-grey color, called polychromatophilic cells. They are very young reticulocytes containing much RNA. Figure 11 compares a polychromatophilic RBC to a smaller, mature RBC on its right. ESRD patients treated successfully with epoetin will have increased numbers of *both* reticulocytes and polychromatophilic cells. This increased number of larger, immature RBCs can cause the mean cell volume (MCV) to increase. The RBC indices may show slight macrocytosis with an increase of the MCV.

Dietary Factors

RBC production requires that all nutritional components be present and in adequate amounts: calories, all essential amino acids, water-soluble vitamins, fat-soluble vitamins, minerals, hormones, enzymes, and iron.

The renal diet is probably the most difficult diet for long-term patient care. Dietary therapy should be a critical concern in the management of the dialysis patient. Unfortunately, the time and energy spent by most dialysis personnel in correcting, assessing, and treatment is minimal. There are no monetary rewards for the dialysis facility which devotes the requisite time to the dietary needs of dialysis patients.

The renal diet is designed to meet the nutritional needs of the patient while limiting foods that produce harmful, waste products.

The individual patient dietary prescription may vary, but the target range for the various restricted food stuffs and liquids remains narrow. The physician should alter this dietary prescription based in the individual patient diagnosis and nutritional needs. However, most attention is not paid to the individual patient, but to the "lab values" that are on the patient's chart.

Table 1: Adult ESRD Diet Prescription

Substance	*Suggested 24 hr Intake*
Protein	1 gm/kg[‡]
Calories	35 kcal/kg[‡]
Sodium	1 - 2 gm
Potassium	1.5 - 3.0 gm
Calcium	1 gm
Phosphorus	0.6 - 1.2 gm
Fluids	1 Liter

‡ per kilogram of lean body weight, see "Protein Prescription" beginning on page 20.

The few patients that learn and adhere to their diet generally feel better, experience a healthier quality of life, have more energy, and tolerate the dialysis treatment with more equanimity, (Table 1).

Protein

Adequate intake of dietary proteins is essential for maintaining body tissue and for body growth. There is no spare protein in the body. Ingested protein is used to build and repair cells or used as fuel.

Amino acids are small compounds that are the building blocks of proteins. Essential amino acids are those which must be ingested and can not be manufactured by humans. Both infants and uremic patients require histidine as an essential amino acid. Uremic patients, require nine (9) essential amino acids, the normal adult only eight (8). Histidine is necessary for red blood cell production.

Animal Protein

Animal protein is protein derived from animal flesh or animal sources, such as:

1   meat
2   fish
3   poultry
4   eggs
5   milk.

Animal proteins are high biological value proteins, they contain an adequate mixture of all the essential amino acids. High biological value proteins are those that allow the body to convert most of the ingested protein into human protein. Whole egg protein has a biologic value of ninety-four percent (94%); dried beans have a biologic value of forty percent (40%).

Vegetable Protein

Vegetable protein comes from plant sources, such as:

1   nuts
2   beans
3   fruits
4   vegetables
5   cereals
6   breads.

Vegetable proteins are low biological value proteins. They contain some of the essential amino acids. If different vegetable proteins are eaten together, such as corn and soybean, all the essential amino acids will be present in that mixture. However the biological value of that vegetable protein mix will still be less than an equal amount of animal protein. The excess protein in that vegetable protein mix will be "burned" and the nitrogen of that protein will be converted to urea; measured as blood urea nitrogen (BUN).

19

Thus, patients who follow a strict vegetarian diet, (and whom eat the same number of grams per kilogram of body weight of protein as non-vegetarians) may have a somewhat increased pre-dialysis BUN as compared to those patients who eat an equal weight of animal protein.

Protein Prescription

Most hemodialysis patients need to eat about one gram of protein per kilogram per day (1 gm/kg/day) of their lean body weight. Lean body weight is an often quoted but little understood classification of body weights. Lean body weight refers to the patient's weight adjusted for age, sex, body habitus, and height according to a chart of values for these variables. The most widely used table in America is the actuarial chart of lean body weights published by the Metropolitan Life Insurance Company.

Lean body weight

The lean body weight of a patient has also been referred to by some investigators as an ideal body weight. Using an estimate of lean body weight to determine protein and calorie need will not worsen obesity nor fail to consider the protein and calorie needs of the underweight, malnourished patient.

Body Mass Index (BMI)

Rather than a chart of idealized body weights for adults, the BMI is used by the World Health Organization (WHO) and a growing number of health-care organizations to assess nutritional status. The BMI is calculated by using the patient's height and weight. The original formula is:

$$BMI = \frac{Weight\ in\ Kilograms}{Height\ in\ Meters\ squared}$$

The formula for those who use pounds for the weight measure and inches for height is:

$$BMI = \frac{Weight\ in\ Pounds\ times\ 703}{Height\ in\ Inches\ squared}$$

The *suggested* BMI range[i] for normal adults in the United States of America (USA) is from nineteen *through* twenty-four (19 - 24). A BMI of twenty-five *through* twenty-nine (25 - 29) is defined as over-weight. BMI values over twenty-nine are defined as obesity. A BMI of twenty-two (22) is very close to the actuarial chart weights for lean body weight or ideal body weight. A BMI of less than nineteen, may mean malnutrition. A table of BMI values using height in feet and inches and weight in pounds is provided as part of this monograph on page 186.

Dry Weight

Lean body weight is not the same as dry weight. Dry weight is an estimation of the weight of a patient without any blood or extracellular volume expansion. It is an estimation of a person's weight in normal fluid balance. No effort is made in estimating dry weight to adjust for patients who maintain their total body water in a water excess state by drinking too much water, who have polydipsia.

Polydipsia and Thirst

There are a number of dialysis patients who have water excess. They have a chronically low pre-dialysis serum sodium. Some of these poor souls were instructed by someone in the distant past to drink eight (8) glasses of water each day to "flush their kidneys." This conscious behavior develops into a habit, and persists when they move on to dialysis therapy. Such patients, more often than not, will be problematic in controlling their blood pressure. Dialysate sodium is now higher than their serum sodium. Their post-dialysis serum sodium is reset *higher*, to a level that causes them to be thirsty. A thirst that is indistinguishable from the thirst of:

1   blood loss

2   hypovolemia

3   iron deficiency

4   water depletion.

i.   Sponsored by the American College of Physicians – American Society of Internal Medicine, November, 1998

They have become compulsive water drinkers; they have psychogenic polydipsia. With the use of epoetin, which can rapidly cause a state of relative iron deficiency as RBC manufacture is markedly increased, patients whom never evidenced excess thirst or polydipsia before may begin to do so. Thirst for water, cold drinks, and ice are classic symptoms of iron deficiency.

High Biologic Value Protein

It is recommended that about seventy five percent (75%) of the total protein intake each day be of high biological value. Most of the high biological value protein is used to make new body protein and produces little urea.

Failure to eat an adequate amount of protein and/or calories results in the body cannibalizing its own protein for energy and to generate new protein.

Unless the patient consumes an adequate amount of the correct protein, calories, and other food stuffs, he/she will enter a catabolic state (when the breakdown of protein exceeds the production of new protein). This is an insidious form of progressive malnutrition.

Protein/Caloric malnutrition should strongly be suspected if the BUN drawn pre-dialysis (before the first dialysis of the week) is less than 60 mg/dL coupled with a serum albumin of less than 3.5 g/dL. Calculate the BMI, if it is less than nineteen (19), the physician and dietitian should be advised. The BMI chart on page 186 should be consulted.

Amino Acid Loss with Hemodialysis

It should be remembered that amino acids are low molecular weight compounds. They are removed by dialysis. One estimate of this essential amino acid loss per dialysis is that of one whole egg or about seven (7) grams of protein.

Calories

Food energy is measured in calories. A food calorie is a large calorie, a kilocalorie. It is that amount of energy that it takes to raise one (1) kilogram of water one (1) degree centigrade.

A calorie is a unit of measure of heat and energy. If all the calories a person ate were converted to energy; a seventy (70) kilogram person eating a one-thousand four-hundred calorie (1,400 kcal) meal would generate enough heat to raise the body's temperature about twenty degrees (20°) centigrade! In a temperate or warm climate, most food calories are directed toward immediate energy and stored energy (fat) production.

Most calories come from non high biologic value protein sources as:

1 fats

2 vegetable protein

3 sugars.

Caloric Prescription

The young adult hemodialysis patient requires about thirty-five kilocalories per kilogram per day (35 kcal/kg/day) of lean body weight. Caloric needs are adjusted *upwards* for those that work physically demanding jobs or for patients below their ideal body weight, and *downwards* for older patients who are less physically active.

Infection, fever, surgery, and other catabolic states increase caloric needs – sometimes to more than double the basal caloric requirements.

Failure to provide the additional calories during these critical times results in muscle wasting and a rapid onset of malnutrition. This situation will result in an increase in the morbidity and mortality of the hemodialysis patient.

Metabolic Free Calories

Non-protein calories or metabolic free calories, are found in fats and carbohydrates (sugar and starches). Free calories come from foods that when "burned," leave little or no waste products in the body that must be removed by the artificial kidney. When starches, sugar, and fats which contain no salts are digested, the principal by-products are carbon dioxide and water. Since carbon dioxide is removed by the lungs and the water of metabolism generated by these free calories has only a small effect on the patient's total body water, these sources of caloric energy are called metabolic free calories.

Salt free fats are an excellent source of calories for hemodialysis patients. Fats provide 9 kcal/gm. Oils, unsalted butter and margarine are examples of these fats.

Sources of sugar include pure sugar, candies, jellies, jam, honey, and complex carbohydrates. These carbohydrates are contained in the starches of low sodium breads, cereals, pasta, and bakery products labeled "Low Salt." Regular bread and bakery products are high in sodium.

Assessing State of Nutrition

Serum Albumin

The serum albumin is the most commonly used indicator of the patient's state of nutrition. The serum albumin *probably* reflects the protein stores in the body and is a ready and simple indicator of the patient's state of nutrition.

Some investigators have complained that since albumin has a long half-life, the serum albumin drawn today actually reflects a clinical state of some days to weeks previously. It is important, therefore to examine the *trend* of the values of the serum albumin levels. A downward trend with a lowering BMI indicates a serious malnutrition problem. A lack of improvement of a low serum albumin indicates lack of adequate nutrition or complicating medical or surgical illnesses. Many inflammatory states may also result in a depression of the serum albumin.

ESRD Albumin Range is Lower

The acceptable range for the serum albumin is 3.5 - 5.5 grams per deciliter (g/dL) for adults without renal failure. The range of serum albumins for dialysis patients, 3.5 - 5.0 g/dL, is lower than the range found in adults without ESRD. It is unusual to see the serum albumin greater than 5.0 g/dL in a dialysis patient though this level is considered normal for an adult. A high pre-dialysis serum albumin in a dialysis patient may be indicative of ECF depletion, commonly called, "saline depletion." If the patient has ECF depletion due to excessive ultrafiltration during dialysis treatment or body fluids loss from gastrointestinal (GI) losses, the patient's Hematocrit (Hct) and Hgb will also be increased.

A low serum albumin (hypoalbuminemia) contributes to edema and shock with usual ultrafiltration during dialysis. Poor wound healing occurs as a consequence of a low serum albumin. Adequate nutrition and a serum albumin of greater than 3.5 g/dL is a mandatory part of adequate dialysis therapy.

Serum Transferrin

The serum transferrin level is another indicator of adequate protein intake and nutrition. A serum transferrin level of 250 milligrams per deciliter (mg/dL or g/L) is considered normal.

Vitamins and Folic Acid

Vitamins and substances that aid those vitamins, are special compounds that accelerate or enhance metabolic processes and chemical reactions in the body.

The ESRD patient may often present to the dialysis unit for his/her first treatment with multiple vitamin and/or folic acid deficiencies. Some drugs, such as Dilantin™, interfere with the absorption and storage of folic acid. Folic acid and vitamin B_{12} are necessary for red and white blood cell production.

For most dialysis patients, it is advisable to prescribe a vitamin B complex mixture, the water-soluble vitamins, plus folic acid.

Vitamin A, D, and E are fat-soluble and not dialyzable. Some over-the-counter multiple vitamins may contain large amounts of these fat-soluble vitamins with inadequate amounts of the water-soluble vitamins and folate.

The use of over-the-counter vitamins or large dosages of vitamins should be avoided. Fat-soluble vitamins, particularly Vitamin A, can cause serious intoxication if used in excessive quantities.

Folic Acid and Homocysteine

Folic acid in amounts over 0.8 milligrams per tablet requires a prescription in the USA. Folate is dialyzable and the amount contained in the non-prescription vitamin B complex tablet, sometimes only 0.4 milligrams, may be inadequate. Folic acid is an important and necessary compound for RBC production. It also is important in reducing the level of an amino acid, homocysteine in the blood. Elevated plasma homocysteine is associated with heart disease and a marker for left ventricular hypertrophy (an abnormally thickened wall of the left ventricle of the heart). Dialysis patients have a high prevalence of elevated plasma homocysteine. Folic acid of 2.5 to 5 mg three times a week, post-dialysis, has been shown to lower these elevated levels of this amino acid[2]. If the dialysis patient is compliant with medications, then a regimen of twice daily folic acid should be implemented. Homocysteine is an amino acid and is dialyzable, but dialysis, by its self, *cannot* correct the elevated homocysteine.

Iron, Transport and Storage

Iron is required for hemoglobin synthesis. Only a small fraction of the iron in the diet or dietary iron supplements is absorbed from the small intestine. Iron is recaptured and conserved by the body during normal RBC breakdown. The total amount of iron in the body is approximately 4 - 5 grams. Sixty five percent (65%) of all iron is incorporated in hemoglobin. Fifteen to thirty percent (15 - 30%) is stored in the form of ferritin. The remaining four percent (4%) is in the form of heme compounds and about 0.1 percent is in combination with the iron transport protein, transferrin. Unless iron is given in large and toxic doses, only a small and limited amount of *oral* iron is absorbed. In children, large doses of oral iron tablets eaten because the tablets were mistaken as candy, have caused iron toxicity.

Transferrin is the plasma protein responsible for iron exchange between tissues. Iron not used to form hemoglobin or myoglobin, combines with a protein called apoferritin to form ferritin. Iron stored in the form of ferritin is called storage iron. When available iron levels in the blood plasma become low, iron is mobilized from ferritin stores and transported as transferrin to where it is needed.

Iron for Erythropoiesis

The serum ferritin and the serum iron transferrin saturation (TSAT) are the best chemical indicators of iron availability. The serum ferritin indicates iron stores. To support erythropoiesis in the patient receiving epoetin, the serum ferritin should be equal or greater than 100 ng/dL. The serum iron transferrin saturation indicates the amount of transferrin iron available for erythropoiesis. To calculate the TSAT, divide the serum iron by the total iron binding capacity. The TSAT should be greater than 20% to avoid iron deficient erythropoiesis. "Relative Iron Deficiency" beginning on page 62, discusses new trends and newer acceptable laboratory values regarding iron therapy.

Hematocrit

In the United States of America (USA), the Hct is the blood test most commonly used to monitor the anemia of dialysis patients. The Hct is the percentage of RBCs in the total volume of the blood sample, (Figure 12). There are two different methods in use to perform the hematocrit test. A blood specimen can be sent to the laboratory for analysis or the test performed in the dialysis setting.

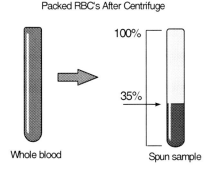

Packed RBC's After Centrifuge

100%

35%

Whole blood   Spun sample

Figure 12 - Hct, a percent of Whole Blood

Hct in the Dialysis Unit

To determine the Hct in the dialysis setting, the patient is first heparinized. Then approximately one-half of a milliliter (½ mL) of blood is drawn from the arterial sleeve of the blood lines at the beginning of dialysis. Or a sample is collected directly from the arterial access prior to connecting the patient to the arterial blood line.

Two micro-capillary tubes are filled with whole blood, sealed, spun in a micro-centrifuge, and then read with a special hematocrit reader. It is imperative to read the Hct test from both tubes immediately after spinning the specimen. Over time, the RBCs tend to de-compact, leading to inaccurate test results.

Note: all microcapillary tubes must be made of plastic to avoid the risk of puncturing oneself with a broken glass micro-capillary tube.

Hcts Sent To The Laboratory

Hematocrits sent to the laboratory require special test tubes with an additive or anticoagulant to prevent the blood from clotting. These tubes commonly contain the anticoagulant EDTA (ethylene diamine tetraacetic acid), which forms a complex with the blood Ca^{++} and prevents the blood from coagulating. The Vacutainer™ system for blood collection uses EDTA as the anticoagulant.

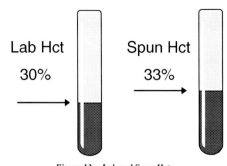

Lab Hct 30%

Spun Hct 33%

Figure 13 - Lab and Spun Hcts

The Vacutainer™ system consists of a plastic tube containing a partial vacuum, a tube holder and a disposable multi-sample collecting needle. The amount of blood to fill these test tubes is approximately 3 - 5 mL. The Vacutainer tube should be at least three-fourths full. It is important to thoroughly and gently mix the additive with the blood after filling the test tube to avoid clotting of the specimen. A partially clotted specimen will yield inaccurate results.

Laboratory Hcts are analyzed using automated hematology instruments. The lab Hcts usually have a *lower* value than centrifuged or spun Hcts by as much as one to five percent (1 - 5%). This is probably due to trapped plasma in the spun Hcts.

Ultrafiltration Effects the Hct

The Hct is typically performed once per week pre-dialysis, usually at the beginning of the week. The Hcts must be done –consistently– before the first, second, or third dialysis of the week in order to be of any value. Patients are generally most edematous prior to the first dialysis of the week. Their Hcts will be the lowest prior to the first dialysis and conversely highest prior to the last dialysis of the week. If Hcts are drawn without regard to the scheduled sequence of dialysis treatment, substantial errors will be made because of this effect of extracellular volume (ECV) on the Hct value.

An average Hct for adult males is forty-seven percent (47%) plus or minus five (±5) or a range of forty-two to fifty-two percent (42% - 52%). The normal hematocrit value for females is forty two percent (42%) plus or minus five (±5) or a range of thirty seven to forty seven percent (37% - 47%).

The difference in the hematocrit between men and women is probably related to the male hormone testosterone. Testosterone stimulates erythropoiesis; it can act in the absence of erythropoietin.

Note: *Always observe gown, glove, and needle precautions when obtaining or handling any blood specimen. See Standard Precautions, Appendix H – Infection Control beginning on page 183.*

Red Blood Cell Indices

RBC indices, or indexes, are calculations first introduced by Doctor Wintrobe to help classify anemias by RBC size and hemoglobin content. Originally, the three (3) RBC indices:

- Mean Cell Volume (MCV)
- Mean Cell Hemoglobin (MCH)
- Mean Cell Hemoglobin Concentration (MCHC)

were calculated from the RBC count, Hgb, and Hct, which were directly measured.

With laboratory automation, the Hct is no longer measured directly, it is calculated. The RBC indices are now calculated using the directly measured:

- RBC count
- Hgb
- Mean Cell Volume (MCV).

The MCV is an important variable in cataloging and understanding the anemias of ESRD. The three (3) types of anemia by RBC size are:

1   Microcytic, smaller than normal RBCs, low MCV

2   Normocytic, normal RBCs, normal MCV

3   Macrocytic, larger than normal, RBCs, high MCV

The two (2)[ii] kinds of Hgb content for RBCs are:

1   Normochromic, normal content of Hgb in the RBC

2   Hypochromic, low content of Hgb in the RBC

ii.   There is no hyperchromic Hgb content of RBCs

Common Types of Anemias Seen in ESRD

Normocytic and Normochromic

- Hypoproliferative anemia associated with ESRD
- Early iron deficiency.
- The MCV is 90 ± 5 fL; MCH is 32 ± 2 pg.

Microcytic and Hypochromic

- Iron deficiency anemia.
- The MCV is < 85 fL; MCH is < 30 pg.

Macrocytic and Normochromic

- Vitamin B_{12} or folic acid deficiency
- Liver disease
- Chemotherapy
- Bone Marrow disease
- The MCV is > 100 fL; MCH is > 30 pg.

"Glossary of Terms" beginning on page 117, contains definitions and formulas for the RBC indices: MCV, MCH, and MCHC.

Complete Blood Count

A complete blood count (CBC) is a group of *screening* blood tests. The CBC is one of the most common blood tests ordered. It determines the number, variety, percentage and quality of the: RBCs, WBCs, RBC morphology, RBC indices, and estimates the platelet count or adequacy. Most CBC tests are done using the Vacutainer system with the anticoagulant EDTA. Table 2, "Complete Blood Count Components," on page 31, lists the components of the CBC.

Blood Groups

There are four main blood groups or blood types. They are A, B, AB and O. Their names are based according to the antigens present or absent on the red blood cell membrane. They are located on the surface of the red blood cell and cause the body to produce antibodies. *Type A* has the antigen A on the red blood cell. *Type B* has the antigen B on the red cells. *Type AB* has both antigen A and antigen B on the red cell. *Type O* has neither the A or B antigen on the red cell. Type O is called

Table 2: Complete Blood Count Components

Test	Symbol
Differential White Cell Count	Diff
Hematocrit	Hct
Hemoglobin	Hgb
Mean Cell Hemoglobin	MCH
Mean Cell Hemoglobin Concentration	MCHC
Mean Cell Volume	MCV
Platelet Count	
Red Blood Cell Count	RBC count
Red Blood Cell indices	
White Blood Cell (WBC) Count	WBC count

a universal donor due to the absence of antigens on the red cell. An O type person can therefore donate blood to all blood groups.

Blood types are either Rh positive or Rh negative. Rh positive blood contains a RBC Rh antigen. Rh negative blood has no antigen present on the RBC.

Blood types are genetically determined. They play a significant role in blood transfusions, tissue and organ transplantation. Blood typing determines compatibility of a donor and recipient for blood transfusions and renal transplantation. An incompatible blood transfusion reaction can be fatal.

All blood donors and recipients are tested for blood types to prevent any transfusions with incompatible blood types. Prior to giving a patient a blood transfusion, two professionals (nurses or physicians) must check and verify that the blood transfusion is for that patient with that specific blood type.

White Blood Cells

A white blood cell (WBC) is also called a leukocyte. WBCs are one of the first lines of defense against both infectious agents and other foreign material. WBCs are motile. They are able to move out of the capillaries toward microorganisms or other injurious substances that have invaded tissues. WBCs are formed *both* in the red bone marrow and in the lymphatic tissue.

The different types, or lineage, of WBCs are: granulocytes, monocytes and lymphocytes. The granulocytes are divided into neutrophils, eosinophils, and basophils. Table 3 "Cellular Elements of Blood" on page 34 outlines the types of WBCs and their different roles.

Figure 14 - Neutrophil

Neutrophils are involved in phagocytosis, (Figure 14). WBCs may destroy microorganisms and foreign particles by ingesting and digesting them; the Latin prefix "phago" means "to eat." Neutrophils are also known as polymorphonuclear cells or "polys." One of their primary purposes is to combat bacterial infections. If there is a break in the skin accompanied with dirt or another foreign body, the neutrophils will be drawn to that area of the skin and attempt to engulf the foreign material. Neutrophils account for approximately 65 - 75% of all WBCs.

Figure 15 - Band neutrophil

Mature neutrophils have a segmented nucleus as shown in Figure 14, normally from two to five (2 - 5) lobes. In cases of inflammation or infection, the bone marrow releases less mature neutrophils with an unsegmented nucleus, as shown in Figure 15. These are band neutrophils. An increased percentage of these cells in the differential WBC is called a shift to the left. Table 4 "WBC Differential" on page 35 indicates the normal level of these cells.

Monocytes are also involved in phagocytosis of foreign matter, (Figure 16). They also combat viruses. They accomplish this by directly interacting with the virus or by production of antibodies to render them harmless. Monocytes account for about 2 - 8% of WBCS.

Figure 16 - Monocyte

Figure 17 - Lymphocyte

Lymphoctyes play a role in antibody formation and the development of immunity, (Figure 17). Lymphocytes respond to the presence of foreign proteins introduced into the body. Antigens are foreign proteins. The antibodies react with the antigen in an attempt to destroy it or render it harmless to the body. The average percentage of lymphocytes is between 20 - 35%. If a patient receives a kidney transplant, the recipients lymphocytes will infiltrate the area around the transplanted kidney. The lymphocytes form antibodies to destroy the foreign cells (transplanted kidney). Immunosuppressive drugs are used to suppress this lymphocyte activity.

Figure 18 - Eosinophil

Eosinophils are associated with allergies and involved in allergic responses, (Figure 18). Eosinophils store a small amount of histamine. An elevation in the eosinophil count is usually a signal that the patient is allergic to something, has an allergic type disease, or is infected by parasites. The typical percentage of eosinophils is between 1 - 4%. Physicians specializing in hay-fever and other allergic disorders may obtain a nasal swab to test for the presence of eosinophils; a positive test indicating a nasal allergy.

Basophils contain histamine and the anticoagulant, heparin. The role of basophils is not clearly understood, (Figure 19). The basophils comprise less than 1% of the total population of WBCs. Possibly the histamine released from damaged cells, brings the anticoagulant to inflamed tissues.

Figure 19 - Basophil

Figure 20 - Platelets

Platelets are also called thrombocytes. Figure 20, shows a group of platelets which have a diameter of about one to two (1 - 2) microns. Platelets play a vital role in hemostasis. Hemostasis is the stoppage of bleeding by a series of events that usually begins with platelet aggregation at the bleeding site. The normal platelet count is between 150,000 to 300,000 per cubic millimeter (mm^3). The average life-span of normal platelets is seven to ten (7 - 10) days. The platelet count in the well dialyzed ESRD patient is normal. But ESRD patients, especially with advanced, untreated uremia have platelets that are less adhesiveness or "sticky." Platelets usually initiate a clotting process when a blood vessel is injured or punctured.

Table 3: Cellular Elements of Blood

Blood Cell	Graphic	Function	Life Span	Time
B Lymphocyte		Antibody immunity	?	
Basophil		Contains Histamine and Heparin	?	
Eosinophil		Allergic Immune response	?	
Erythrocyte		Transport O_2 and CO_2	100 - 140	days
Monocyte		Immune Response	3	days
Neutrophil		Phagocytosis	7	hours
Platelets		Blood Clotting	7 - 10	days
T Lymphocyte		Cellular immunity	?	

WBC Count

The test to determine the number of WBCs is the WBC count. The WBC count measures the total number of white blood cells. The normal WBC count is usually between 5,000 to 10,000 per cubic millimeter (mm^3). The WBC count includes a differential count. The differential count, lists the percentage and kinds of the different types of WBCs, (Table 4). The sum of the percentages of different types of white blood cells will total one hundred percent (100%). Often, the differential count can be clinically significant and important.

The physician may order a WBC count when assessing the patient for a possible infection in the dialysis setting. An elevation of the white blood count above normal may indicate the presence of an infection, a pyrogen reaction, stress, or use of steroid type hormones. A complete blood count (CBC) may be ordered to assess the differential count of WBCs and the Hct.

A healthy person who develops a systemic bacterial infection, will show an increased WBC count in a matter of four to eight (4 - 8) hours. In patients that are ill, aged, or immunosuppressed, the WBC count may not show an increase for up to 24 - 48 hours. This situation can occur in non-ESRD patients who are malnourished, debilitated or just chronically ill. Dialysis patients who are ill, under-dialyzed, or aged may show a delayed WBC count elevation.

Table 4: WBC Differential

Cells	Count/mm^3	Percent
Neutrophil	6,000	60%
Neutrophil, band	500	5%
Eosinophil	300	3%
Basophil	100	1%
Lymphocyte	2,500	25%
Monocyte	600	6%

Obtaining an Accurate WBC Count

An accurate WBC count and differential can only be obtained *before* a dialysis treatment. The WBC count drops almost immediately after beginning dialysis. The post-dialysis WBC count may reflect changes induced by the dialysis treatment.

As dialysis therapy is started, the WBCs, specifically the neutrophils, migrate to and sequester in the lungs causing a drop in the WBC count of up to fifty to eighty percent (50 - 80%). These sequestered WBCs probably never return to the blood stream. The normal or near normal WBC count seen post-dialysis is due to immature WBCs released from the bone marrow or due to the release of marginated WBCs (WBCs attached to cells lining blood vessels). About fifty percent (50%) of WBCs in the blood are marginated and not represented by the WBC count. Thus, the post-dialysis WBC count may be normal. But the *differential* WBC count will show a shift to the left of neutrophils (*see* "Band neutrophil" on page 32) and *incorrectly* suggest a serious bacterial infection. The many dialysis practitioners who draw post-dialysis CBCs should not do so.

The reason for this pulmonary sequestration of WBCs is not understood. It is thought to be due to complement activation between the dialyzer membrane and the blood. It may be associated with a decrease in the arterial oxygen concentration. By the conclusion of the dialysis treatment, the WBC count, generally, returns to the pre-dialysis value. Because of these issues, WBC counts probably should not be taken during the dialysis treatment, for the results are likely to be inaccurate or misleading.

Blood Coagulation

The term coagulation means clotting. Blood, normally, is continuously clotting to repair microscopic defects or injuries in the blood vessel walls. These clots serve as temporary plugs to stem the leak of blood. The clots dissolve over time and are replaced by normal cells, such as the lining cells of blood vessels, or with scar (fibrous tissue) which occurs with AV fistula venipuncture to perform hemodialysis.

Lysis means to decompose or dissolve. In a normal healthy adult, the continuous clotting and repair process of microscopic defects in the blood vessel lining is normal, physiologic, and causes no tissue build up in the blood vessels. In the presence of vascular disease, such as coronary artery disease, the clotting process in diseased blood vessels leads to tissue formation, narrowing of the blood vessel lumen and eventual vessel occlusion.

Clotting Process

Injury to the blood vessel lining or contact of blood with a foreign surface initiates the clotting process. Immediately, platelets clump together to form a plug at the site of injury. The platelets release a substance called platelet factor 3 that accelerate the activity of other blood coagulation factors. These events lead to the actual clot formation. Platelet factor 3 aids in the eventual dissolving of the clot. Uremic patients have impaired platelet factor 3 function. The clotting process occurs as a continuous process, but is depicted as a series of three stages, (Figure 22).

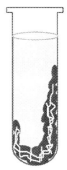

Figure 21 - Fibrin clot

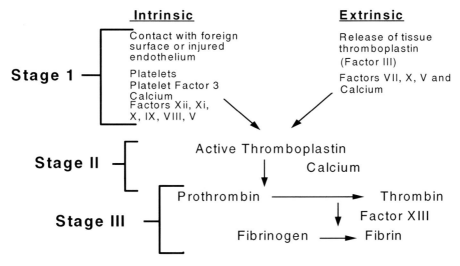

Figure 22 - Three stages of Clotting

Blood proteins, prothrombin and fibrinogen participate in the clotting process. Prothrombin converts to thrombin. Thrombin converts fibrinogen, a soluble plasma protein, into fibrin. Fibrin is a whitish threadlike, stringy material which forms a mesh, a framework for the blood clot. When blood clots in a glass test tube (Figure 21), the clot will eventually contract and shrink leaving a fluid above and around the clot. That fluid is serum. Serum is plasma minus fibrinogen and prothrombin. The fibrinogen is now fibrin and part of the blood clot.

Hemostasis

Hemostasis means to stop the blood from flowing in a vessel or to stop the bleeding. Hemostasis depends on:

1   the ability of normal blood vessels to contract (reduce in size) and retract (draw back) when injured

2   the ability of platelets to form plugs in the injured blood vessels

3   the presence of plasma coagulation factors

4   the stability of the blood clot.

Dialysate and Plasma

Dialysate solution or dialyzing fluid is a non-sterile aqueous electrolyte solution that is *similar* to the normal levels of electrolytes found in extracellular fluid. Dialysate solution is a near isotonic solution, with an osmolarity of approximately 300 ± 20 milliosmoles per liter (mOsm/L). Osmolarity refers to a known number of particles, ionized or non-ionized in a known volume. To assure patient safety, the osmolarity of dialysate must be close to the osmolarity of plasma. The osmolarity of plasma is 280 ± 20 mOsm/L.

For dialysis, the composition of the blood plasma (not the blood water) is the isotonic standard. The intravenous solution we use and call normal saline (0.9% NaCl), has an osmolarity of 308 milliosmoles per liter. It is *slightly* hypertonic to normal blood plasma.

IV Hypertonic NaCl

Some dialysis facilities inject very hypertonic (23.4%) NaCl solutions IV to treat muscle cramps. The blood in the blood line downstream from this injection immediately darkens probably because the RBCs are severely crenated and some may hemolyze.

Table 5: Comparing Dialysate & Blood

Substance	Dialysate, Low	Dialysate, High	Units	Blood, Low	Blood, High
Sodium	135	145	mEq/L	135	145
Potassium	0	4	mEq/L	3.5	5.5
Calcium	2.5	3	mEq/L	4.5	5.5
Magnesium	0.5	1	mEq/L	1.5	2.5
Chloride	100	115	mEq/L	95	105
Bicarbonate	30	40	mEq/L	22	28
Dextrose	0	200	mg/dL	80	120

Hypertonic solutions have a higher osmolarity than body fluids. Exposing the blood to a hypertonic solution may cause shrinkage, crenation, of the RBCs. Hypertonic solutions increase the osmolarity of plasma. The osmotic pull, causes water to leave the cells, reducing the interstitial and intracellular fluid. As water leaves the cells, the cells shrink; they crenate. Exposing a patient's blood to a hypo-

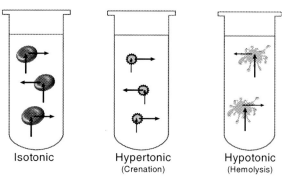

Isotonic   Hypertonic (Crenation)   Hypotonic (Hemolysis)

In comparison of solutions, the larger arrows indicate greater movement of water in or out of the red blood cell.

Figure 23 - RBCs & Osmolar Effects

tonic solution may cause hemolysis. Plain or tap water is a hypotonic fluid. A solution with a lower osmolarity than body fluids will transfer fluid to the interstitial and intracellular fluid compartments. The osmotic pull is greater within the cell; as water enters the cells, they hemolyze and rupture releasing hemoglobin into the plasma.

Infection Control

Infection control in the dialysis setting focuses on:

1 the patient
2 dialyzer
3 dialysate
4 treated water
5 access to the circulation.

Bacteria and viruses account for most infectious problems in dialysis. An understanding of infection control techniques is required for the safety of patient's and staff.

A blood-borne pathogen is an organism that can be transferred from one person to another from exposure to an infected patient's blood and/or body fluids. The major communicable, blood-borne pathogens seen in dialysis units are:

1 hepatitis B virus (HBV)
2 hepatitis C virus (HCV)
3 human immunodeficiency virus (HIV).

Because of a series of outbreaks of HBV, precautions to prevent the transmission of HBV in dialysis centers were published, originally in 1977, by the Centers for Disease Control and Prevention (CDC).

HBV incidence, prevalence, and transmission in American dialysis units has declined to such a low level that a few cases in one facility are reported by the CDC as an outbreak. Though more serious, major blood-borne pathogens other than HBV, are not as stringently regulated by CDC policies as HBV.

Of substantial concern to the dialysis community are the recent development of antibiotic resistant bacteria:

1 vancomycin resistant enterococci (VRE)
2 methicillin-resistant staphylococcus aureus (MRSA)
3 vancomycin intermediately resistant to staphylococcus aureus (VISA).

Dialysis patients often acquire these infections in the hospital (nosocomial) and bring them into the out-patient dialysis unit after discharge.

To protect health-care workers and patients from exposure to blood-borne pathogens, the CDC and the Occupational Safety and Health Administration (OSHA) have mandated the use and implementation of universal/standard precautions.

Universal Precautions

A standard for universal precautions was developed in 1987 by the CDC. The standard was developed in an to attempt to prevent transmission of common, serious blood-borne pathogens, such as HCV and HIV. The concept of universal precautions, considers blood and certain body fluids of *all* patients as potentially infectious for blood-borne pathogens. Universal precautions mandates that all body fluids are treated as potentially hazardous.

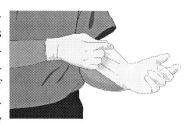

Figure 24 - Always Glove

*Note: HCV is the most common viral hepatitis seen in ESRD patients. The CDC has written about alarmingly high and serious long-term morbidity and mortality due to HCV based on their "unpublished data." The only substantial and **published** study[3] comprising a forty-five (45) year follow-up in healthy adults does not support this; showing a very low liver-related morbidity and mortality.*

The following is extracted and paraphrased from CDC documents, "Universal precautions are intended to prevent parenteral, mucous membrane, and non-intact skin exposures of health-care workers to blood-borne pathogens. In addition, immunization with HBV vaccine is recommended as an important adjunct to universal precautions for health-care workers who have exposures to blood....

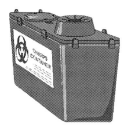

Figure 25 - Always Dispose Sharps

Universal precautions addresses needle and sharps disposal, hand-washing, cleaning, disinfecting and sterilizing, protective barrier precautions in dialysis to prevent skin and mucous membrane exposure when handling all blood and body fluids to protect non-intact skin….

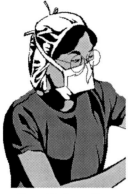

Figure 26 - Protect Face

The use of protective barriers reduce the risk of exposure of the health-care worker's skin or mucous membranes to potentially infective materials (blood, body fluids containing visible blood, and other fluids to which universal precautions apply). Examples of protective barriers include gloves, gowns, masks, and protective eye-wear or face shields. Gloves should reduce the incidence of contamination of hands, but they cannot prevent penetrating injuries due to needles or other sharp instruments. Masks and protective eye-wear or face shields should reduce the incidence of contamination of mucous membranes of the mouth, nose, and eyes."

Standard precautions were published by the CDC in 1996 to replace universal precautions. Dialysis units should incorporate the features of these guidelines. These strategies are effective against the transmission of HBV, HIV, and bacteria such as VRE. Health-care workers must be conscientious about adhering to the infection control guidelines and practices.

The most important rule is proper *handwashing* especially between each patient visit, and after removing your protective gloves.

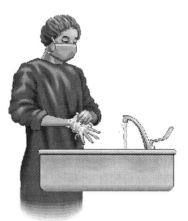

Figure 27 - Must Wash Hands

Note: *For information from the CDC concerning infection control precautions for dialysis units, see "Infection Control" beginning on page 183.*

Anemia and Uremia

A nemia, –derived from the Greek– means "without or no blood." Since "no blood" is incompatible with life, the word anemia actually means a reduction in the concentration and number of circulating RBCs below that found in normal subjects.

Major Function of RBCs

The major function of RBCs is to carry O_2 to all cells in the body and retrieve CO_2 from these cells. Anemia results in less oxygen transport. This cellular hypoxia causes many signs and symptoms. Severe anemia causes the heart to beat faster and increase its output of blood.

Anemia or a deficiency of RBCs is due to:

1   inadequate red blood cell production
2   blood loss
3   abnormal destruction of RBCs
4   and, a combination of abnormalities.

Uremic Anemia

Almost all patients with ESRD are anemic before starting chronic dialysis. This is commonly called "uremic" anemia. The proper term is: hypoproliferative anemia; a lower than normal manufacture and production of RBCs. This uremic anemia is often due to a combination of factors including a decreased production of the hormone, erythropoietin.

Hypoproliferative Anemia

There are several kinds of common anemias that are called hypoproliferative anemia. They are anemias caused by:

1   erythropoietin deficiency
2   iron deficiency
3   inflammatory diseases and states

4   uremia

5   other minor types.

It's important to remember that uremic anemia often consists of the first four (4) diagnoses in the above list.

Assessment of Anemia

It is important to draw the blood sample to assess the dialysis patients' anemic state pre-dialysis. With the usual amount of ultrafiltration, the Hct post-dialysis will be increased. In some cases with large amounts of ultrafiltration, the Hct can increase quite substantially, (Figure 28). The assessment of a patient's anemia should include *both* the testing of blood and an assessment of how the patient feels.

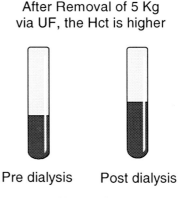

After Removal of 5 Kg via UF, the Hct is higher

Pre dialysis   Post dialysis

Figure 28 - Pre and post Hct

Anemic signs and symptoms depend upon many factors, including the patient's physiologic age. Thus, patients with the same chronological age and with the same degree of anemia will show markedly *different* clinical signs and symptoms. The common laboratory tests used to measure anemia are:

1   RBC count

2   Hct

3   Hgb.

Hematocrit

ESRD patients have Hcts ranging from a low of twelve to a high of fifty-four percent (12% - 54%) before starting maintenance hemodialysis. Since predialysis use of human recombinant erythropoietin (epoetin) is not universal, patients may begin their very first dialysis with a very low Hct. It is imperative to obtain a predialysis Hct in these patients as their ability to withstand even modest amounts of ultrafiltration will be seriously compromised if their Hct is under 20% and disastrous if as low as 12%.

Low Hcts in America

Recent American studies indicate that forty five percent (45%) of the dialysis patients may have hematocrits of less than 30% and eight percent (8%) of patients demonstrate severe anemia with hematocrits of less than 25%. Figure 29 summarizes the sales of epoetin alfa in the USA for a five (5) year period, from 1991 to 1995, as reported by Amgen in their annual report for 1995. IV iron was not available in part of 1991 and part of 1992. The epoetin alfa sales were four hundred million US dollars in 1991 and approached one billion US dollars at the end of 1995. The average Hct in those five (5) years only increased about two percent (2%). These data came from Amgen's and the United State Renal Data System (USRDS) annual reports. This graph suggests that spending a billion dollars a year for a miracle medication *without proper education* may have little effect.

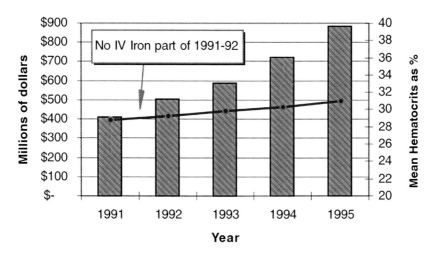

Epogen Sales - Amgen's 1995 Annual Report

Figure 29 - Epoetin sales versus Hct

Pre and post dialysis Hct

Typically, Hcts are drawn weekly. The Hct should be drawn pre-dialysis. Ultrafiltration of ECF, also called ECV, leads to an increase in Hct post-dialysis from that of the pre-dialysis level. The Hct must be drawn under the same clinical conditions each time in order to compare Hcts and adjust epoetin dosage.

Dilutional Anemia

The Hct must be corrected for ECV expansion in the dialysis patients. With ultrafiltration during dialysis, the post-dialysis Hct should be higher than the pre-dialysis value. The pre-dialysis Hct is measured when the patient is volume expanded. The degree of volume expansion is seen by assessing:

1   patient's weight

2   evidence of edema

3   elevation of neck vein pressure

4   sitting and standing blood pressures.

The average ESRD patient's weight pre-dialysis is almost always higher than their estimated dry weight. The blood pressure will usually be above normal in most patients who have evidence of excess extracellular fluid volume.

Hct, Better for Assessing ECV

Each liter of ECV excess will *lower* the Hct about one to three (1 - 3) points; each liter of ECV loss will *raise* the Hct a similar amount. Some writers have mistakenly concluded that the Hgb is a better test for anemia because the Hgb changes *less* with extracellular volume expansion. Both Hct and Hgb change to the same degree with extracellular volume expansion and depletion. The Hct shows more dramatic changes with ECV changes because it's value is three (3) or more times the Hgb value.

Dry Weight

Dry weight is the colloquial term used to describe the status of a patient with no fluid excess in their interstitial and plasma compartments. It is a clinical *guess* of the patient's true and normal ECV. The assumption is made that the post-dialysis Hct more accurately reflects both the patient's *true* Hct and dry weight. There is a substantial correlation between excess ECV and hypertension, the post-dialysis blood pressure most often is low or normal.

The Hct is the percentage of RBCs in the total volume of blood. Since ultrafiltration removes plasma ultrafiltrate the Hct, percentage of plasma proteins, and Hgb values are all increased post-dialysis.

Hemoglobin

The normal blood hemoglobin ranges between twelve to sixteen grams per deciliter (12 - 16 g/dL). The hemoglobin normally reflects the Hct value by a ratio of about three (3) to one (1) {Hct/Hgb 3:1}. Because of how Hgb is measured in the laboratory, in some unusual cases, the measured Hct will decrease without a similar change in the Hgb. This can occur with massive intravascular hemolysis. Hgb is a measure of RBC heme pigment in blood while the Hct is a measure of packed RBCs classically determined by centrifuging a blood sample.

Tissue hypoxia can occur without evidence of anemia. Methemoglobinemia, caused by drugs or toxins, renders RBCs unable to carry oxygen efficiently. With methemoglobinemia, neither the Hct or the Hgb accurately reflects the RBCs ability to carry and release oxygen to the tissues. Signs and symptoms of hypoxia occur with methemoglobinemia.

ESRD patients dialyzed with water contaminated with nitrates (due to fertilizer or bacterial growth) have developed methemoglobinemia. Sodium *nitrite* ingestion has also been reported to cause methemoglobinemia.

Hgb or Hct – Gold Standard

Hgb measurement is replacing the use of the Hct in many American dialysis clinics. The Hgb is a more stable and probably a more accurate test than the Hct measurement, which is *calculated* from two other measured variables.

The Hgb value is closely allied to the Hct. One can use the ratio of 3:1 to 3.3:1 to calculate the Hct from the Hgb. One must be aware that the *normal* ratio of Hct to Hgb is not 3:1 but closer to 3.3:1. Health Care Financing Administration (HCFA) requires that a value for Hct be attached to all Medi-Care bills for dialysis patients. HCFA uses the Hct/Hgb ratio of 3:1. Epoetin usage may increase the Hgb/Hct ratio.

47

In well dialyzed patients, a Hct/Hgb ratio may be *higher than 3.1*, more on the order of 3.2:1, thus the *calculated* and reported Hct is *lower*. With the HCFA reimbursement cutoff for epoetin of 36.5%, this calculation error allows the reporting of lower Hcts.

Reticulocyte Count

Reticulocytes normally comprise about one percent (1%) of the total RBC count. This is consistent with the normal loss of one percent (1%) of RBCs per day in a steady state.

In evaluating the bone marrow's response to an anemia, the reticulocyte count should be corrected, downward, for the anemia; doing so will give the observer a better idea of how the bone marrow is responding to the anemic drive to make RBCs. One formula for the corrected reticulocyte count is:

$$Corrected\ Reticulocyte\ Count = Reticulocyte\ Count \times \frac{Patients\ Hct}{Normal\ Hct}$$

If the Hct is 22.5%, the reticulocyte count is 3%, and a normal Hct of 45% is selected for the formula: the corrected reticulocyte count is 1.5%, barely above or normal. The reticulocyte count has a substantial margin of counting error, with normal reticuloctye counts up to 1.7%. A corrected reticulocyte count of 1.5% in the presence of anemia indicates an abnormally low RBC production response given that degree of anemia.

The absolute reticulocyte count is another formula used to estimate the reticulocyte production. The reticulocyte count, as a percent, is multiplied by the RBC count (in mm^3 or $10^{12}/L$) to give the reticulocyte count per microliter (μL) of blood. If the reticuloctye count is 1% and the RBC count is five million (5,000,000/mm^3), the absolute reticulocyte count is fifty-thousand (50,000/(μL).

This second formula is:

$$Absolute\ Reticulocyte\ Count = Reticuocytle\ Count \times RBC\ Count$$

Normal reticulocytes are called one day reticulocytes as they only exist as reticulocytes for one day in the blood, becoming mature RBCs in that time period. But with the treatment cocktail of epoetin, intravenous iron, multivitamins, better nutrition, and –hopefully– adequate dialysis therapy; the reticulocytes exit the bone marrow sooner and last two or three days in the blood. This is called a *reticulocyte shift*.

The reticulocytes are no longer one day reticulocytes and a *second* correction factor must be used to account for the reticulocytes that last two to three days in the blood before becoming mature RBCs. This is the reticulocyte production index formula. It should be used to correct for the reticulocytes in the blood that last more than one day. This third formula is:

$$Reticulocyte \ \ Index \ = \ Reticulocyte \ \ Count \times \frac{Patients \ \ Hct}{Normal \ \ Hct} \times \frac{1}{2}$$

and uses the "fudge factor" one-half (½) to reduce the reticulocyte count. A low, less than two percent ($< 2\%$) reticulocyte index points to low bone marrow RBC output and a hypoproliferative anemia such as seen in ESRD.

With epoetin treatment, an elevated reticulocyte count is the first clear evidence of increased RBC production. If the patient is suspected to be unresponsive to epoetin, the corrected reticulocyte count will confirm this unresponsive state.

Adequacy of Dialysis

Adequacy of dialysis contains many elements of patient care that can not be identified nor determined by any one finding or lab test[4,5].

Adequacy of Dialysis and Erythropoiesis

The benchmark of adequate hemodialysis is the ability to maintain a satisfactory Hct in an ESRD patient without the need for blood transfusions. Prior to 1989 and the ability to treat dialysis patients with epoetin, many nephrologists[6] had from twenty-five to fifty percent (25 - 50%) of dialysis patients with stable, albeit, low Hcts, ranging from the low twenties to the high forties (20s - 40s). Those who preferred to treat patients with peritoneal dialysis lectured that though their patients had slightly lower serum albumins, they *all* had higher Hcts!

High BUN Causes Platelet Dysfunction

Despite much research, there are no identifiable uremic toxins which cause morbidity and death of the ESRD patient. A high blood urea causes only minor signs and symptoms. Investigators who use urea, or BUN, and formulas to measure or equate adequacy of dialysis treatment with urea have caused us, unfortunately, to focus on a minor issue.

Doctor William J Johnson when he was chief of nephrology at Mayo Clinic in Rochester, Minnesota, reported in 1972[7] how he successfully hemodialysed three (3) ESRD patients with *urea* in the dialysis bath. Urea has a molecular weight of sixty (60), BUN makes up less than one-half (½) of that molecular weight. *"Examples of Conversion to SI Units" beginning on page 182* discusses urea and BUN. Doctor Johnson maintained pre-dialysis blood ureas in these ESRD patients of one-hundred to three-hundred (100 - 300) mg/dL. Only at the 300 mg/dL levels did he observe signs and symptoms associated with high blood urea.

Urea is Not a Uremic Toxin

One incapacitated patient who had to be maintained on bed rest with persistent headache, vomiting, and pleurisy (inflammation of the lining of the lungs causing painful breathing) was begun on chronic hemodialysis therapy with a dialysis bath urea of two-hundred to three-hundred (200 - 300) mg/dL. Over several dialyses, this patient's strength returned, headache, vomiting and pleurisy remitted. She was discharged from the hospital in about two (2) weeks. All three (3) patients had increased bleeding from around the vascular access sites, nose bleeds, and easy bruising with minor trauma. High blood urea interferes with platelet factor 3.

A 1979[8] paper describing the neurologic effects of uremia written by Doctor P J Dyck a Mayo Clinic neurologist, showed that a high blood urea is associated with some neurologic difficulties. These are the only studies by the same group that dealt with urea toxicity with *prospective clinical studies* in ESRD patients.

Markers for Adequacy of Dialysis

Adequacy of dialysis includes an assessment of the patient's need for erythropoietic substances and the treatment needed for the patient to manufacture blood. The most successful dialytic care should be that which requires:

1   no medicines to treat hypertension
2   no epoetin
3   no emergency intervention for hyperkalemia
4   no emergency intervention for volume overload and congestive heart failure

5   no repeated vascular access surgeries by a surgical team not committed to excellence of care

6   no intervention for poor wound healing, malnutrition, or low serum albumin

7   no need to assess URR or Kt/V as the previous markers render a dialysis dose marker unnecessary and counterproductive. Dialysis dose markers take away focus from the real issues; the continuous assessment of quality of patient care.

Doctor Bernard Charra

Doctor Bernard Charra's dialysis program in Tassin, France fits most of the above markers for adequacy of dialysis. No American nephrologist or dialysis company has followed his example stating that no American would tolerate eight (8) hours of hemodialysis three (3) times a week.

Doctor Charra's patients have a 5% annual mortality[9]. His patients are dialyzed using the 1970's "Seattle System" of a two layered modified Kiil dialyzer with blood flow rates of about 200 mL/min. His patients have a Kt/V of about 2.0, higher for the patients who weigh less, and almost no patients require anti-hypertensive medication. With high-efficiency dialyzers, and a blood flow rate of 350 mL/min, his dialysis treatment can be accomplished in about four and one-half to five (4 ½ - 5) hours.

Number of Medications, a Gold Standard?

If one were to attempt to focus on any single, simple marker of adequacy of dialysis, it would –possibly– be the number of medications that the patient *routinely* required. This does not mean that the patient would not intermittently need IV iron or antibiotics or other medications. A gold standard might be the number of medications as a fraction of the number two (2); as there are two (2) necessary medications. Thus, the patient who takes a B and C complex multi-vitamin (with an adequate amount of folic acid) and a second oral medication to control hyperphosphatemia, would have an adequacy factor of 100%. The dialysis patient, who uses ten *routine* (10) medications, would have an adequacy factor of (2/10) or twenty percent (20%).

Signs and Symptoms of Anemia

Symptoms

Anemic patients show a variety of clinical signs and symptoms. Usually, the symptoms are proportional to the degree of anemia and the age of the patient. The average age of ESRD patients has increased substantially and aged patients do not tolerate anemia with the alacrity of youth. For patients of equal age and health status, patients with a hematocrit of 20% are usually more symptomatic than patients with a hematocrit of 30%. Severely anemic patients exhibit generalized fatigue. They move slowly and are short of breath with little exertion. The most common complaint is weakness. Rarely excessive thirst for cold drinks or ice occurs. This thirst and craving for cold and ice may reflect profound iron depletion.

Headaches, dizziness, angina (chest pain), and dyspnea (shortness of breath) with exertion are other complaints. Some may complain of: generalized coldness, loss of appetite, insomnia, depression, and sexual disinterest.

Signs

Skin blood flow decreases with age. The flush and bloom of youth gives way to the sallowness of age. A search for skin changes associated with anemia requires that mucus membranes be examined for pallor. Iron deficiency as a partial cause of "uremic" anemia causes nails to be brittle and change in shape from the normal convex shape to a concave spoon shape. Resistant anemia may be due to malnutrition with hypoalbuminemia. While examining the patient's nails for signs associated with iron deficiency, hypoalbuminemia can be diagnosed by the presence of opaque white bands of the finger nails called Muehrcke's bands or lines.

Anemia contributes to hypotensive episodes during the dialysis treatment due to vigorous –and appropriate– ultrafiltration. These hypotensive episodes are difficult or impossible to treat. Progressive weight gain, with edema leading to heart failure can occur in elderly patients with inappropriate anemia.

Each year, the average age of the American dialysis population increases. Each year these elderly patients become less tolerant of a less than optimal Hct.

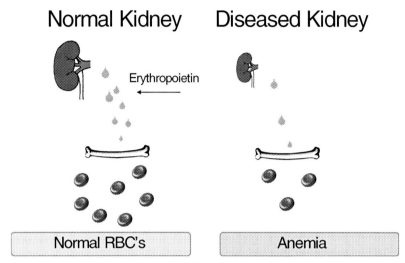

Figure 30 - Erythropoietin Production

Decrease Production of Erythropoietin

Figure 30 depicts the relationship of kidney, bone marrow, and erythropoietin in producing RBCs. As renal failure progresses, the kidney's ability to produce erythropoietin diminishes. The degree of damage to the kidneys usually correlates with the degree of anemia in the ESRD patient.

Although the number of RBCs decreases, the RBCs are normal in size and color. The RBCs are normocytic and normochromic. Normocytic means normal in size. Normochromic means normal in color. Iron deficiency causes microcytic, hypochromic RBCs.

RBC Survival

The normal, average life span of RBCs is about one hundred and twenty (120) days. The average dialysis patient has a RBC survival about one-half (½) normal or sixty (60) days. The RBC survival in these individuals ranges from one-third (1/3) normal to normal.

The cause of shortened survival of the RBCs is thought to be mild hemolysis related to the "sick cell" concept. Patients with diminished renal function have accumulation of yet unidentified toxins leading to the notion of a generalized toxic state or "sick cells."

Hemolysis

Hemolysis is the destruction of RBCs. The RBCs swell, burst, and release their hemoglobin into the surrounding fluid. Hemolysis can occur as a direct result of the dialysis treatment.

Acute hemolysis

Acute hemolysis can result in a dramatic decrease in the patient's Hct and create a medical emergency. The most frequent causes are:

1   chloramines, and other water disinfectants

2   cold sterilants or disinfectants in the dialyzer or fluid delivery system

3   hypotonic dialysate

4   mechanical hemolysis or injury of RBCs from occluded or kinked hemodialysis blood lines

5   over-heated dialysate.

Causes of Hemolysis

Chloramines

Chloramines are a group of compounds used to disinfect drinking water. They are made by reacting chlorine with ammonia. Chloramines are cellular oxidants. They cause red blood cell injury.

Chloramines can cause different levels of RBC injury:

- hemolysis
- hemolytic anemia
- methemoglobinemia.

Depending upon dose and patient susceptibility, hemolysis can occur rapidly or over a prolonged time period. A small amount of chloramine causes methemoglobinemia and characteristically stippled RBCs called Heinz bodies.

Methemoglobinemia effects the hemoglobin portion of the red blood cell, decreasing its ability to carry oxygen.

Attempting to view a Wright stained RBC slide to see Heinz bodies is futile. The RBC blood film must be prepared with the stain crystal violet or brilliant cresyl blue for these rounded clumps to be seen, (Figure 31). They are believed to be denatured hemoglobin; thus indicating RBC injury.

Figure 31 - Heinz bodies

Unoxygenated blood is darker than oxygenated blood. Classically, the patient is fatigued, Short of Breath (SOB), and cyanotic.

Cyanosis can not occur in a severely anemic patient as cyanosis requires that about five (5) grams of hemoglobin be converted to the methemoglobin state. Thusly, cyanosis may be absent in the very anemic dialysis patient.

Special laboratory tests show the presence of Heinz bodies and methemoglobinemia. Exposure of the patient's blood to large amounts of chloramines causes acute hemolysis. The hematocrit decreases rapidly, the patient becomes acutely ill, and the patient may die.

Chloramines in dialysate water occur because of improper removal during dialysis water treatment and inadequate water testing in the facilities. A municipal water supplier may suddenly add chloramines or other RBC oxidents without alerting dialysis facilities. This has happened in California on at least three (3) occasions.

Methods of water treatment to eliminate chloramines include:

1 carbon tanks pre water treatment
2 ascorbic acid added to the dialysate bath.

The use of chloramine test kits to assess chloramine levels in water for dialysis is mandatory and will prevent this problem. The State of California mandates chloramine testing every patient shift.

Nitrates

The presence of nitrates in drinking water occurs more commonly in farming communities. Contamination of water by bacteria and fertilizers is the source of these contaminants.

Nitrate poisoning in dialysis patients was first described as the well water syndrome. This occurs with home dialysis patients whose source of water is local well water. Nitrates in dialysis water cause methemoglobinemia and hemolytic anemia. Nitrate water contamination can also occur in urban settings.

Copper and Zinc

Copper poisoning in dialysis patients is commonly due to the presence of copper plumbing in the water treatment system and/or water distribution system in the dialysis unit. Water used in a dialysis unit is processed to be almost pure, containing only dissolved CO_2 from the air. That water is mildly acidic. Acidic water flowing through copper plumbing will dissolve minute quantities of copper from that plumbing.

Copper poisoning can cause hemolysis, pancreatitis, and liver damage. Plumbing consisting of galvanized iron can cause high levels of zinc in dialysis water. The zinc can leach from galvanized iron piping. Zinc poisoning causes nausea and vomiting, fever, and anemia.

Plumbing materials used in the water treatment system and water distribution system in dialysis must be non-reactive with purified water. Brass, copper, aluminum and zinc (galvanized iron) are not to be used in hemodialysis plumbing.

Acceptable materials include polyvinyl chloride (PVC), non-pigmented poly-propylene, stainless steel, and glass. The most common type of plumbing material used in dialysis is PVC.

Osmolar Injury

Exposing blood to a hypotonic solution causes osmolar injury to the cells. The difference in the solute concentration between the solution and blood causes water to move into the cells. Exposure to hypotonic dialysate is the most common cause of hemolysis during dialysis and can be fatal within a few minutes.

Hypotonic dialysate

Hypotonic dialysis causes generalized swelling of body cells and, if severe enough, acute hemolysis. The patient may suffer from cerebral edema and may have seizures.

Low conductivity of the dialysate is the most common type of conductivity alarm. Most commonly, the dialysate concentrate container empties during the dialysis treatment. If the dialysis machine goes into the bypass mode, there is no harm to the patient. If the internal or external low conductivity limits are not adjusted properly and/or the machine does not go into the bypass mode, the patient's blood is exposed to hypotonic dialysate.

Each machine should be checked *pre-dialysis* to insure that there is adequate dialysate concentrate in the container. The dialysis staff should not rely on the conductivity meter to monitor dialysate concentrate supplies.

Hemolysis Due to Heat

If the dialyzing fluid equals or exceeds 108° F or 42° C, hemolysis will occur. Certain model fluid delivery machines are equipped to use heat disinfection. Heat disinfection of the dialysis fluid path is performed with water heated to almost boiling temperatures, about 185° F or 85° C.

After heat disinfection, it is critical to allow the machine to properly cool down prior to patient use. Machines using heat disinfection should have a built in safety feature that will not allow the machine to go into the dialyze mode or allow the blood pump to operate until the temperature has dropped well below 42°C.

Cold Sterilants or Chemical Disinfectants

Chemical disinfection may be done with a variety of chemicals. Residual cold sterilants or disinfectants used to disinfect water lines, fluid delivery machines and reprocess dialyzers may cause hemolysis.

The most common chemical disinfectants are:

1   sodium hypochlorite (household bleach)
2   formaldehyde
3   peracetic acid.

To prevent any hemolysis, proper tests should be done for residual cleaning agents or disinfectants.

Residual Testing

Reprocessed dialyzers must have residual safety tests performed after priming, *prior* to starting dialysis. All dialyzers require labeling, indicating the presence of the chemical disinfectant and the need for residual testing.

Chemical disinfection of the dialysis machine and water distribution system is done *after* the patients are disconnected from dialysis machinery. A complete rinse cycle of the dialysis equipment must be done before and after chemical disinfection. During and after chemical cleaning, all machines should be clearly labeled indicating the presence of the chemical disinfectant and the need for residual testing.

Table 6: Common Residual Safety Tests

Chemical	Name of Test	Residual in ppm
Bleach	Chlorine Reagent Test Strip	0.0 ppm
Bleach	Hemastik®[‡]	50.0 ppm
Chloramine	La Mott Chloramine Test	0.01 ppm
Formaldehyde	Clinitest®[‡]	50.0 ppm
Formaldehyde	Formasure®	3.0 ppm
Peracetic Acid	Residual Renalin® test strip	0.0 ppm

[‡] not recommended - not as sensitive as other safety tests

A Timed Rinse is Not Adequate

A timed rinse is *not* adequate to insure all the cleaning agents have been removed. Failure to test for residual cold disinfectants and cleaning agents, may result in silent hemolysis. Table 6 lists common chemicals, their tests, and the least level of the compound that can be identified by the test.

Mechanical Injury of RBCs

Mechanical injury to RBCs can cause hemolysis during hemodialysis. A 1996 article[10] reported ten (10) episodes of hemolysis, over a one (1) year period. There was one (1) patient death. Despite intensive investigation no cause was determined until kinking of the arterial blood line was noted with an episode of hemolysis. The kinking was between the blood pump and the arterial drip chamber. A subsequent hemolytic event was associated with kinking after the blood pump but before the inlet to the dialyzer. These obstructions did not cause a pressure monitor alarm as there were no arterial pressure monitors used in this dialysis facility.

The CDC reported an outbreak of hemolysis in May 1998, which affected thirty (30) patients in three (3) states. There were two (2) deaths. These episodes were caused by a manufacturing flaw in the blood tubing sets. Marked narrowing at the arterial drip chamber caused mechanical lysis of the RBCs.

Hemolysis Signs and Symptoms

The amount and intensity of exposure to the hemolytic agent will dictate the degree of non-specific signs and symptoms.

Signs

1 shortness of breath

2 nausea and/or vomiting

3 sweating (diaphoresis)

4 hypotensive shock

5 death, in severe cases.

Symptoms

1 back pain

2 tightness in chest

3 chest or abdominal pain

4 headache.

In mild acute hemolysis, the blood in the venous blood line may become *lighter* in color giving a cherry-pop appearance. With severe and sudden hemolysis, the blood can *darken* in the venous blood line and change from bright red to dark red.

If hemolysis is identified in a symptomatic patient, dialysis must be *stopped* immediately. Clamp the arterial and venous blood lines, turn off the blood pump and place the machine in the bypass mode.

Do Not return the hemolyzed blood to the patient. The hemolytic agent may be present in the extracorporeal circuit. The hemolyzed blood is high in potassium. This is an emergent condition. Assume the hemolysis may continue; hospitalization and observation is usually mandated.

Lab Analysis for Hemolysis

An immediate assessment of acute hemolysis can be done in the dialysis facility. Take a blood sample from the one of the blood lines and centrifuge it. If there is substantial hemolysis, the plasma will be pink tinged. Obtain a "Stat" hematocrit. With acute hemolysis, and the presence of pink plasma (Figure 32), the Hct will be lower than the patient's previous Hct.

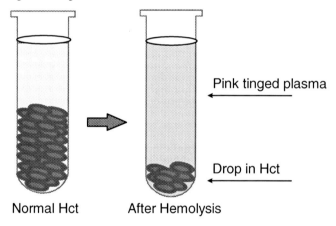

Figure 32 - Hemolyzed Blood

If the patient has not eaten, non-hemolyzed plasma is clear and straw colored. Additional lab data should show the presence of Heinz bodies, pink plasma, and a lowered serum haptoglobin. As little as hemolysis of ten (10) milliliters of blood will tinge the plasma pink for a few hours.

Classic medical studies on acute hemolysis were done on patients with normal renal function which excrete this unbound plasma hemoglobin quickly; the plasma color returns to its normal straw color in a few hours, (Figure 33). There is very little information on how long plasma hemoglobin remains in the dialysis patient after massive intravascular hemolysis. In addition to the direct evidence of

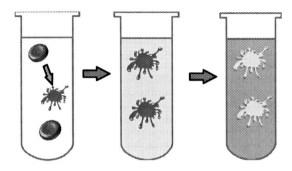

Figure 33 - RBCs & Hemolysis

intravascular hemolysis, RBC breakdown causes an increases in:

1   creatine phosphokinase (CPK)

2   lipase

3   serum amylase.

Iron Deficiency and Epoetin

Iron deficiency is the most common cause of anemia in the USA. The true importance of abundant iron therapy was not widely appreciated when epoetin was first used. In normals, erythropoietin levels in the blood is in milli-units per mL (mU/mL), from 9 to 26 mU/mL. Natural, native erythropoietin has a concentration at maximum of 26 U/L. The distribution volume of erythropoietin is similar to blood volume, about five (5) liters[11].

Epoetin and Pharmocologic Dose Levels

Thus, the total amount of circulating normal erythropoietin is about one-hundred and thirty (130) units. Commonly, dialysis patients are given IV epoetin in doses of 50 to 150 U/kg of body weight. Giving epoetin to a seventy (70) kilogram patient at a dose level of 150 U/kg is a total dose of 10,500 units of epoetin. This translates to a dose that is *a hundred times* the physiologic level of erythropoietin levels seen in normals whom are not anemic.

True, anemic individuals will increase their native erythropoietin production ten to hundreds (10 -100s) of times the normal levels in response to tissue hypoxia, as shown in Figure 35 "Erythropoietin response" on page 81. But the breakpoint where normal erythropoietin is increased is about a Hgb of 12 and the physiologic elevation of erythropoietin for anemia at or just below a Hgb of 12 may be up to ten (10) times the normal level. That would mean a total amount of circulating erythropoietin of 260 U/L. In a seventy (70) kilogram person that is a total *dose* of epoetin of 1,300 U, or 18 U/kg of body weight given IV twice a day. If this reasoning is accepted, the epoetin dose is an indicator of adequacy, or inadequacy, of dialysis. "Adequacy of Dialysis and Epoetin" on page 80 gives further information about this issue.

Relative Iron Deficiency

Table 7: Lab Values for Iron Deficiency and Excess

Test	Increased Iron	Normal	Iron Depletion	Iron Deficiency
Ferritin	High	Normal	Low	Very Low
Plasma Iron	High	Normal	Low	Very Low
RBCs	Normal	Normal	Normal	Microcytic
Transferrin	Low	Normal	Normal	High
% Transferrin Saturation	High	Normal	Low	Very Low

After IV epoetin, the amount of readily available stored iron may not be enough to support the dramatic increase in erythropoietic demand. Iron deficiency, inadequate dialysis, and malnutrition are the major factors in persistent anemia in the ESRD patient. Iron is an important component in the formation of the protein heme of RBCs. Iron deficiency inhibits RBC production. The lab values associated with various iron states, from iron excess to severe iron depletion are outlined, (Table 7). Note that the Transferrin Saturation (TSAT) is a ratio and composed of two other values the plasma iron and the transferrin (Transferrin Iron

Binding Capacity). The plasma iron can vary by as much as 30% depending on the time of day drawn. A daily variability of blood level of a substance is called a diurnal variation. Plasma iron concentration has a substantial diurnal variation. The plasma ferritin is a much more reliable indicator of body iron than the TSAT.

Acute Phase Reactants

Investigators[12] have proposed that a serum ferritin level of less than 100 nanograms per milliliter (ng/mL or μg/L) and/or a percentage Transferrin Saturation (TSAT) of less than 20%, are/is clinical evidence of iron deficient erythropoiesis. However, transferrin and ferritin are acute phase reactants. Their blood levels change –in opposite directions– in response to inflammation, infection, and other bodily insults.

Ferritin, an Acute Phase Protein

A low plasma ferritin is the gold standard of iron deficiency. Only two other clinical conditions will *lower* plasma ferritin:

1 hypothyroidism
2 ascorbate (Vitamin C) deficiency

Ferritin is an acute phase protein and its blood level *increases* in response to fever, chronic inflammatory diseases, acute infections, rheumatoid arthritis, et cetera.

Negative Acute Phase Proteins

Unlike ferritin, transferrin blood levels decrease with the same conditions that increase ferritin. Transferrin, like albumin, is a *negative acute phase protein*. Transferrin levels *increase* with iron depletion and *decrease* with iron overload *if the patient is not ill*. Transferrin, like albumin, is also a marker of adequate protein nutrition and will *decrease* with malnutrition. Since the plasma iron level is diurnal and varies by as much as 30%, and the transferrin level is effected by so many different conditions, it seems ill advised to compare a TSAT (plasma iron divided by transferrin) to the present gold standard for bio-available iron, plasma ferritin.

Higher Standards for Iron Adequacy

Newer, *higher* standards for iron assessment are sought by some, choosing higher serum ferritins of 300 - 500 ng/mL and TSAT of 25 - 35%. These higher values are based on a theory of "relative unavailability of stored iron for RBC manufacture." This concept is termed functional iron deficiency.

Iron Deficiency Definitions

Iron deficient states for the ESRD patient can be defined as:

Absolute Iron Deficiency, Gold Standard

A stringent definition[1], the lack of visible or stainable iron in an adequate sample of red bone marrow.

Absolute Iron Deficiency by Lab Tests

1   serum ferritin less than 15 ng/mL with[12],

2   a TSAT of less than sixteen percent (16%)

ESRD Iron Deficiency

1   serum ferritin less than 100 ng/mL with[12],

2   a TSAT of less than twenty percent (20%)

Relative or Functional Iron Deficiency

1   serum ferritin greater than 100 ng/mL with[12],

2   a TSAT of less than twenty-five percent (25%),

3   *and*, evidence that both ferritin and TSAT have been *decreasing* with epoetin therapy,

4   *and*, Hct response to epoetin has been blunted or stopped, necessitating an increase in epoetin dosage,

5   *and*, administration, by IV, of 500 mg or more of iron,

6   *resulting in*, an increase of Hct or a reduction of epoetin dosage

Functional Iron Deficiency?

Adequacy of dialysis was briefly discussed, on page 49. The term functional iron deficiency needs to be carefully considered and not used casually. The term functional, as applied to medical terminology, means without causation or etiology. The diagnosis of functional iron deficiency can only be made when the following conditions are excluded:

1   inadequate dialysis therapy

2   acute phase protein changes, *see* page 63

3   Vitamin C deficiency, *see* page 72

4   all important diseases and conditions associated with anemia as discussed in "Diagnosing Functional Iron Deficiency" below.

Table 7 on page 62 gives the values and findings of normal individuals with various iron storage states. These values reflect: no illness, no infection, no malnutrition, and no acute phase protein changes. The casual diagnosis of functional iron deficiency without regard to a careful evaluation of the patient will lead to increasing the doses of powerful and highly reimburse able drugs, epoetin and iron; but without correction of the true illness.

Diagnosing Functional Iron Deficiency

Functional iron deficiency may be suspected when an ESRD patient's Hct does not improve in two to four weeks with usual epoetin dosage that formerly increased the Hct.The following issues, diseases, and conditions are the common causes of non or hypo responsiveness to epoetin therapy. To determine the cause and correct hypo responsiveness to epoetin, the following must be ruled out:

1   no drugs which interfere with epoetin such as the commonly used anti-hypertensive drugs called Angiotensin Converting Enzyme (ACE) inhibitors[13]

2   no infection or inflammation

3   no recent surgery

4   no renal bone disease, especially no high blood aluminum level

5   no systemic disease such as lupus erythematosus, multiple myeloma, rheumatoid arthritis, or other systemic illnesses which are associated both with renal failure and anemia

6   a normal bone marrow!

7   no hemoglobinopathy

8   no under-dialysis

9   no malnutrition.

10   no glucose 6 phosphate dehydrogenase (G6PD) deficiency, *see* page 76

11   no vitamin C, folic acid, B_{12}, B complex, or other vitamin deficiencies.

Causation of Iron Deficiency in ESRD

Fortunately, if the ESRD patient's general needs are taken care of, iron deficiency occurs in dialysis patients for two (2) basic reasons:

1   failure to replace iron stores

2   blood loss.

Dialysis patients normally experience bleeding problems. Bleeding can result from excessive anticoagulation therapy with:

1   heparin

2   aspirin compounds

3   oral anticoagulants, such as Coumadin.

Bleeding can result from capillary fragility or abnormal platelet function. Patients can experience bleeding from any part of the body:

1   gastrointestinal (GI) tract

2   nose

3   genitourinary (GU) tract

4   menstruation

5   hemorrhoids

6   breaks in the skin.

Blood Loss

Blood loss results from the dialysis therapy for several reasons. The many reasons include:

1   blood sampling

2   retention of blood in the dialyzer and blood tubing post-dialysis

3   clotted dialyzers and blood lines

4   ruptures of dialyzers

5   inattentive (sloppy) nursing technique

6   excessive bleeding from AV fistula needle sites post-dialysis.

66

Blood sampling for laboratory tests is probably the most overlooked contribution to blood loss. Repetitive and un-necessary blood drawing contributes to blood loss and increases the exposure of personnel to blood borne infections!

Blood sample volumes vary from five to one hundred (5 - 100) milliliters per week, (Table 8). Residual blood in the dialyzer post-dialysis can vary from five to fifty (5 - 50) milliliters per treatment. Failure to rinse the dialyzer properly with adequate amounts of normal saline while discontinuing dialysis contributes to anemia.

Table 8: Estimate of Blood Loss per year

Amt mL	Frequency	Blood Test	Yearly Total
5	each dialysis	Serum K^+, Hct, et cetera	780
16	per month	Blood chemistry panel, etc	192
16	every 3 months	Hepatitis screening, et cetera	64
15	each dialysis	Residual blood in dialyzer, blood lines, and bleeding from fistula needle sites	2,340
Total mL			3,376

Between blood sampling and residual blood in the dialyzer, conservative estimates of blood loss each year is about three thousand three hundred and seventy six (3,376) milliliters of whole blood per patient. This is equivalent to a normal healthy adult donating about seven (7) pints of blood per year. This is a flagrant disregard for patient welfare and should be an embarrassment to all.

The above estimate of blood loss does not include:

1 GI bleeding
2 *prolonged* bleeding from fistula needle sites
3 blood loss due to careless nursing technique.

Why Conserve the Patient's Blood?

It is critical for all health care workers to treat the patient's blood as a precious and potentially infectious commodity. It has been argued that this attention to conservation of the ESRD patient's blood is unnecessary, even silly, given that epoetin can correct the uremic anemia quite handily. This widespread attitude is to be abhorred; it is incorrect. Blood loss is:

1 protein loss

2 iron loss

3 vitamin loss

4 essential amino acid loss

5 a vehicle for transmission of blood borne diseases

6 culture media for floor, wall, and counter surface bacteria.

Blood specimens should be taken only when necessary. Blood samples need to be taken in minimum quantities for testing. Meticulous methods must be used by all team members during procedures to minimize blood loss.

Techniques must be employed to maximize red blood cell return to the patient when terminating dialysis. This is done by using adequate amounts of IV saline to rinse back RBCs in the blood lines. Iron depletion occurs with blood loss. All of the above mentioned situations contribute to iron deficiency.

Correction of Iron Deficiency

Iron deficiency can be corrected by administering iron preparations to the dialysis patient. Iron preparations are available for oral or intravenous use. Both treatment options present potential difficulties. Oral iron preparations can be slow in correcting iron deficiency and potentially ineffective. Intravenous preparations produce more rapid results, but they pose potential allergic hazards to the patient.

Oral iron preparations and doses vary according to physician orders. The problems with oral iron preparations vary. The most common problems are:

1 slow or poor absorption

2 GI intolerance.

The extensive use of phosphate binders interferes with iron absorption in the GI tract. It advisable that oral iron preparations not be taken at the same time as phosphate binders. GI problems from oral iron therapy include:

1 constipation

2 diarrhea

3 dark stools (simulating GI bleeding)

4 nausea

5 epigastric and chest pain.

To reduce these side effects:

1 decrease doses

2 take iron between meals with snacks

3 increase frequency of doses.

To increase oral iron absorption in the GI tract, some physicians recommend that ascorbic acid be taken at the same time as oral iron.

Patient Non-Compliance

Patient non-compliance with all oral medications, even those without the substantial side effects of iron, is a principal cause of oral iron therapy failure.

IV Iron

Elemental iron given IV, without a compound to bind and complex it, is toxic. Iron is complexed to different compounds and available for IV use as:

1 iron dextran

2 iron saccharate

3 iron gluconate

The IV doses vary widely. A common dose schedule of iron dextran is fifty to one-hundred (50 - 100) mg given for five (5) dialysis treatments for a total dose of 250 to 500 mg of iron complex. Some programs use 50 mg once a week until the ferritin exceeds 700 to 800 ng/mL. Hematologists, treating non ESRD patients for iron deficiency as out-patients, may use much larger single IV doses.

IV infusion of medication carries the risk of hypersensitivity reactions or anaphylactic reactions. A pre-infusion test dose of one drop (0.05 mL) of iron dextran is recommended to rule out any allergic response by the patient.

 Note: A serious anaphylactic reaction may be successfully treated if diagnosed early. The BP must be monitored during any infusion of IV iron and the patient observed for any signs and symptoms of an allergic or anaphylactoid reaction.

An anaphylactic reaction occurs as a result of the introduction of a foreign substance in a person that has been *previously sensitized* to that foreign substance. The body's reaction can range from mild to severe. The symptoms can be severe enough to produce serious shock, even death, if emergency treatment is inadequate. The adverse drug reaction is normally evident within a few minutes after beginning the IV infusion.

Test Dose of Iron Dextran

Though a test dose can range from one tenth to one half of a milliliter (0.1 - 0.5 mL) of the iron dextran; it is recommended to use one drop (0.05 mL) as the test dose. This test dose is given as an intravenous (IV) push prior to the therapeutic dose. The instructions that accompany these medications recommend a waiting period of forty five (45) minutes to sixty (60) minutes. In clinical practice, these recommendations are rarely followed. Evidence of a reaction occurs within a few seconds to minutes of the test dose. Doses and methods of administration of iron dextran vary widely among dialysis facilities:

- most facilities will give the test dose only once, at the beginning of each series of five (5) doses of iron dextran.
- this may be the common practice but we have seen two (2) different patients that demonstrated allergic reactions to the iron dextran in the **middle** of a five dose series.
- the results of iron therapy is monitored by following the serum ferritin and transferrin saturation.
- some dialysis facilities require that an emergency drug cart be available at the patient bedside before giving the test dose.
- rarely, the physician asks to be present when test doses are administered.

Anaphylactic Reaction

Many of the signs and symptoms of an anaphylactic reaction (or an anaphylactoid reaction) are related to the release of histamine from mast cells. Histamine causes constriction of smooth muscles of the upper and lower airway and vasodilation of arterioles and capillaries.

Signs and symptoms of a mild reaction are:

1   itching
2   tightness or a "lump" in the throat
3   hoarseness
4   difficulty breathing
5   back or chest pains
6   urticaria or hives.

With a severe reaction the patient can demonstrate some or all of the above, and:

1   a sudden drop in BP
2   severe shortness of breath
3   wheezing
4   violent cough
5   convulsions
6   loss of consciousness
7   respiratory and cardiac arrest.

Treatment of Anaphylaxis

If an adverse drug reaction is suspected, *stop* the infusion! Implement the emergency standing orders to treat anaphylaxis.

Cardiopulmonary resuscitation may be required. Vasopressor agents such as epinephrine, steroids, and IV antihistamines may be ordered and given. Nasal oxygen should be started.

Vitamin Deficiencies

RBC production requires –among other compounds– folic acid, vitamin B_{12} and iron. Vitamin deficiencies in ESRD patients, though easily avoidable, are often overlooked.

Folic Acid Deficiency

One of the original investigators isolated this vitamin from spinach and gave it the name folic acid. Folate is an ester or salt of folic acid. Folic acid deficiency is sometimes called folate deficiency. Folic acid deficiency may be due to inadequate intake of foods restricted in dialysis diets, such as spinach, and other green leafy vegetables.

Folic acid is a complex of several related small organic acids. It is water soluble and dialyzable. Folic acid is lost through the dialysis procedure. Without supplementation, folate deficiency will occur in a ESRD patient because of diet and dialysis loss. Some prescribed drugs may interfere with the absorption and storage of folic acid, adding to the problem of folic acid deficiency.

The usual regimen for dialysis patients includes a multiple vitamin capsule of B-complex vitamins, vitamin C and folic acid. All are needed for protein and RBC manufacture. These over-the-counter pills can only contain a maximum of 0.8 mg of folic acid, an amount that may be insufficient for the ESRD patient, *see* "Folic Acid and Homocysteine" on page 25.

Vitamin C Deficiency

Vitamin C, ascorbic acid, is a necessary and essential vitamin for ESRD patients. The ESRD patient's diet should be supplemented with oral vitamin C. Vitamin C is involved in absorption of dietary iron, essential in maintaining capillary integrity and in wound healing. Unfortunately there is no simple test for *minimal* vitamin C deficiency. It should be given as a supplement to all ESRD patients unless there is an expressed contraindication. Like any important substance, a little may be "not enough," and a lot may be "too much." Large doses of vitamin C have been associated with oxalate kidney stones in individuals with normal renal function and calcium oxalate deposits in ESRD patients[14].

If the ESRD patient has a pending diagnosis of functional iron deficiency, it may be a vitamin C deficiency. Patients diagnosed as having functional iron deficiency, have been successfully treated with IV Vitamin C *alone*[15] (no additional IV iron or epoetin).

Osteitis Fibrosa Cystica

Osteitis fibrosa cystica is a bone disease. Its name is defined by what one observes through the microscope. There are bone cysts, bone fibrosis, bone destruction and repair giving a pattern of abnormal bone architecture. One of the main causes of this disease state is an abnormally elevated parathyroid hormone (PTH).

This disease state may have an inhibitory effect on erythropoiesis as the red bone marrow –which produces RBCs– is replaced by fibrous tissue. There is less blood producing bone marrow and less stem cells for epoetin to act on.

Aluminum Toxicity

Medical care always involves trade offs. Correcting or treating one condition commonly introduces side effects or causes a brand new disease. In ESRD patients, aluminum related osteomalacia may result from efforts to control and prevent an abnormally elevated PTH. Aluminum bone disease is an excellent example of this phenomenon. The aphorism, "First, do no harm," should underpin all actions of those in the healing arts. Treatments that induce other illnesses or side effects worse than the original disease should be avoided.

Aluminum toxicity can occur from improperly treated water used for dialysate. Much more commonly, aluminum toxicity is due to systemic absorption of aluminum containing antacids. The anemia of aluminum toxicity may be confused with the anemia of iron deficiency for both produce a microcytic anemia.

Proper water treatment to remove aluminum and use of non-aluminum containing antacid therapy may correct this bone disease and anemia. Administration of chelating agents such as desferrioxamine mesylate can reverse the microcytosis. These chelating agents will also chelate iron.

RBC Suppression

A blood transfusion quickly –but only temporarily– raises the Hct. Transfusion therapy suppresses erythropoiesis. This effect seems to be more dramatic with multiple units of blood given at one time as compared to a single unit transfusion. Erythropoiesis suppression is only important for those patients who do not require epoetin, but maintain their Hct by endogenous erythropoietin. These patients can become dependent on blood transfusions to maintain their Hct.

Blood transfusion therapy is not without risk. Blood borne viral infections, especially HCV, bacterial contamination, and anaphylactic reactions should give one pause when contemplating routine blood transfusions to support a dialysis patient's RBC count.

Hypersplenism

Hypersplenism is a disease state due to an enlarged spleen which –abnormally– traps normal white and red blood cells. The spleen lies in the left upper abdomen below the diaphragm, (Figure 34).

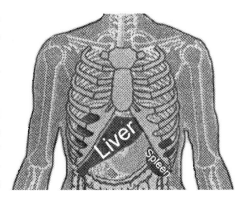

Formerly, hypersplenism was identified and treated in ESRD patients. With the advent of epoetin therapy, it is probably under and misdiagnosed. A careful history and physical examination of the patient has given way to dependency on laboratory data –alone– to diagnose patient illnesses.

Figure 34 - Liver & Spleen

The enlarged spleen can almost always be palpated. With the trapping of RBCs in the spleen, the anemia is accompanied by a low WBC count and low platelet count, pancytopenia. Pancytopenia findings may be present in the patient's weekly and monthly laboratory data, but they are oft times ignored. Hypersplenism accentuates hemolysis and shortens RBC survival. Splenectomy usually results in a remarkable improvement of the anemia.

Short History of Epoetin

- Richard Bright an English physician, in 1836, described anemia as a complication of chronic renal failure. In 1863 a French physician, Dr. Jourdanet, showed the relationship between tissue oxygenation and RBC production.

Doctor Jourdanet made the observation that chronic hypoxia led to polycythemia. Polycythemia is an excess of red blood cells. The body's response to low levels of oxygen in high elevations is to produce more RBCs.

- In 1953, Doctor Erslev and his colleagues of Jefferson Medical College made rabbits anemic by bleeding them. The plasma of the anemic rabbits, injected into normal rabbits, stimulated erythropoiesis. The plasma from these anemic rabbits contained the hormone, erythropoietin.
- In 1977, Doctors Miyake, Kung, and Goldwasser were successful in purifying erythropoietin from the urine of patients with aplastic anemia.
- Doctor Fu-Kuen Lin and others isolated the gene for human erythropoietin in 1983.
- Amgen®, a biotechnology company in Thousand Oaks, California developed the manufacturing techniques of recombinant human erythropoietin (rHuEPO) for human use. Their first recombinant human erythropoietin was named epoetin alfa.
- The first human clinical trials for epoetin alfa were conducted in 1985 in Seattle, Washington by Doctors Joseph W Eschbach and John Adamson. The first clinical trials took place at the Northwest Kidney Center.
- The human clinical trials led to approval by the FDA for epoetin (Epoetin alfa) in 1989 and its clinical use beginning that year.

Treatment of Anemia

The effective treatment of the anemia of dialysis patients may require several modes of therapy, drugs, and diet. If treatment does not produce the desired response rather quickly, more extensive investigation is mandatory.

Androgen Therapy

Before the advent of epoetin, androgen therapy was a mainstay in some centers for the long term treatment of anemia in hemodialysis patients. If reimbursement for epoetin is an issue, androgen therapy may be considered.

Androgen therapy is the use of a synthetic version of the male hormone testosterone. Testosterone can stimulate erythropoiesis in the absence of erythropoietin. The effects of this androgen therapy are slow, and take several months.

One of the common androgens in use to correct anemia is nandrolone decanoate (Deca-Durabolin®). It is given by intramuscular (IM) injection. The dosage in women is 50 - 100 milligrams per week, and in men, 100 - 200 milligrams per week. Another preparation, testosterone propionate tends to be given mainly to men. Though it is preferable to administer these IM injections on off-dialysis days to avoid hematomas or bleeding problems from anticoagulation therapy, this is often impractical and inconvenient for the patients.

Androgen therapy can cause unwanted side effects in both women and men. The side effects can be numerous. Side effects for women include:

1   acne

2   facial hair

3   voice deepening

4   baldness.

Lower total weekly dose can decrease these side effects. Psychological intolerance to these side effects may outweigh the improved Hct. Though reported in the medical literature, male priapism is rare. Priapism is an abnormal, painful and continued erection of the penis.

For androgen therapy to be effective, it is essential that the patient have adequate intake of protein, calories, folic acid and adequate iron levels. Androgen therapy is uncommon in America.

Prior to Administration of Epoetin

Each patient should have a full and careful evaluation before beginning any drug therapy to correct anemia. If the patient is iron depleted, under-dialyzed, has elevated serum aluminum levels associated with aluminum bone disease, or is malnourished, anemia drug therapy will not correct those maladies nor the anemia associated with them.

The patient evaluation should include:

1   serum ferritin

2   serum transferrin and transferrin saturation

3   serum albumin

4   standing pre-dialysis blood pressure

5   estimation of ideal body weight

6   pre-dialysis serum potassium

7   URR or Kt/V values

8   list of other medications which may impair erythropoiesis or inhibit vitamins or other substances needed for erythropoiesis.

9   history, physical, and Review of Systems (ROS) for other causes of anemia such as:

    a: a heredity hemoglobinopathy

    b: drug induced anemia

    c: hemolysis due to an RBC enzyme lack such as glucose 6 phosphate dehydrogenase (G6PD) deficiency. An unstable variant of G6PD deficiency is present in about eleven percent (11%) of black males in the USA. Blacks comprise about forty-percent of the ESRD population. G6PD deficiency, which can induce hemolysis after a single dose of an oral drug such as acetaminophen[i], should have generated more than *one* reported case of G6PD deficiency in ESRD patients... it hasn't.

The serum ferritin should be at least 100 ng/mL and the transferrin saturation at least 20%. The blood pressure should be controlled by medication or judicious use of ultrafiltration prior to therapy. The blood pressure may increase with epoetin therapy. Careful monitoring of the blood pressure is essential.

Description of Epoetin alfa

Epoetin alfa is a glycoprotein and has similar, if not identical, biological effects as human erythropoietin. The molecular weight is about 34,000 daltons. It is formulated as a sterile, colorless, liquid for subcutaneous or intravenous injection. It contains human albumin, probably, to prevent its absorption onto the glass vial. It must be kept in a refrigerated (not frozen) state. This drug requires refrigeration at 36° to 46° degrees Fahrenheit. The vials should not to be frozen. Violent shaking may inactivate the drug.

---

i.   acetaminophen, mild oral analgesic compound used alone or in combination with other drugs. Commonly used in American dialysis units as Tylenol®.

Epoetin alfa is available in one (1) mL single-dose, preservative-free vials containing in Units/mL:

- 2,000
- 3,000
- 4,000
- 10,000
- 40,000

or two (2) mL multi-dose, preserved* vials containing in Units/mL:

- 10,000

or one (1) mL multi-dose, preserved* vials containing in Units/mL:

- 20,000.

*1% benzyl alcohol as preservative in water for injection.

All vials are color-coded to help prevent medication dose errors.

Given IV, epoetin alfa has a half-life ranging from four (4) to thirteen (13) hours. A *half-life,* or T one-half, or t½, is the amount of time it takes to remove, metabolize or inactivate *half* the amount of the initial dose of medication.

Epoetin

Epoetin is a correct and generic name for the class of compounds known as human recombinant erythropoietin. There is more than one of these compounds. Epoetin alfa was the first Federal Drug Administration (FDA) approved epoetin. Epoetin alfa is often referred to by American workers as EPO, its short-hand name. Another recombinant human erythropoietin preparation, epoetin beta, is available for treatment of non-ESRD patients in the USA. Epoetin beta is manufactured by Chugai-Upjohn, Inc and is used outside the USA for ESRD patients. These two epoetins are not identical[18].

Epoetin alfa is a man-made hormone. Chinese hamster ovarian cells are genetically modified by insertion of the gene that manufactures human erythropoietin. A culture of these mammalian cells are grown in glass containers in a specially constructed facility under sterile conditions. The "liqueur" from these cells contains the hormone erythropoietin which is collected and purified. Recombinant means artificially combined (recombined). Epoetin alfa is the only recombinant human erythropoietin permitted for use by ESRD patients in the United States as of this writing.

Epoetin directly stimulates erythropoiesis, increasing the reticulocyte count within seven to ten days (7 - 10). A Hct increase follows within two to four (2 - 4) weeks. Epoetin can be given intravenously during the saline rinse-back; at the end of hemodialysis.

Epoetin, End of Dialysis?

Epoetin alfa is not dialyzable to any significant degree; it's molecular weight is 34,000 daltons. One study in 1995 suggested that epoetin could be given at any-time during the dialysis procedure using high-flux dialyzers and suggested that epoetin was not absorbed to the dialyzer hollow fibers. There were no follow up studies by this author to fully elucidate this preliminary observation.

The original package insert of 1989 from Amgen, stated that epoetin must be given at the end of the dialysis treatment. The latest package insert[17] is somewhat different from the original and states that epoetin alfa, "may be administered into the venous line at the end of the dialysis procedure...." This language implies that epoetin can be given earlier in the dialysis procedure.

Most units have not altered how they give this drug though it creates a rushed and disorderly atmosphere during the end of the dialysis session.

Removing the patient from dialysis should be a time that is ordered, calm, and rea-soned. Some dialysis units have changed their epoetin administration to reflect the non-dialzability of the hormone and administer epoetin sometime during the last hour of dialysis, to perform a safer dialysis procedure.

Subcutaneous Epoetin

Epoetin can be given subcutaneously (SC). Some, not all, studies indicate that epoetin given SC is as effective and can be given as a lower weekly dose than IV epoetin[18]. IV epoetin has a t½ of four to thirteen (4 - 13) hours. Subcutaneous epoetin has a lower peak blood concentration, is less bioavailable than IV epoetin, but has a much longer t½. IV epoetin is 100% bioavaiable (its physiological avail-ability, or the proportion of the administered dose which is absorbed into the bloodstream). Despite SC epoetin's lower bioavailability, the longer t½ of SC epoetin and the resultant sustained erythropoietic stimulus may lead to as much as a thirty percent (30%) reduction of total weekly dose of epoetin.

It should be stressed that this potent drug, by any form of administration, will not be effective if the patient's nutritional requirements are not met. The patient must have adequate iron stores, be adequately dialyzed, and not have any nutritional factors that prevent normal erythropoesis. Since SC epoetin is sometimes required in doses of *over* one milliliter, dialysis anticoagulant therapy becomes important to avoid subcutaneous bleeding from this injection. The issue of excessive heparin is reviewed under "Heparin Half-Life" beginning on page 97.

Indications and Usage

Epoetin alfa, since its introduction in 1989, has become the mainstay in the treatment of the anemia of chronic renal failure. It effectively decreases the need for blood transfusions. It is not a substitute for emergency blood transfusions or for immediate correction of severe anemia. It is not a substitute for determining the adequacy of dialysis for each individual ESRD patient.

Adequacy of Dialysis and Epoetin

In the past five (5) years, we have seen a small population (five percent (5%) of four-hundred and fifty-one (451) ESRD patients) who began dialysis therapy requiring epoetin for months. These patients have maintained their Hct at or above thirty-eight (38) percent for over a year *without* epoetin. The Hcts of a few patients have continued to climb to as high as fifty (50) percent causing concern about erythrocytosis, (*see* page 89). All of these epoetin-independent patients are without evidence of severe hypoxia or the clinical diagnosis of polycystic kidney disease. Both of the previous conditions are known to result in Hcts in ESRD patients that are increased without the use of epoetin.

A normal Hct in ESRD patients, maintained without epoetin, is a physiological marker of adequate dialysis care. The ability of an ESRD patient to make blood and maintain their Hct without the use of human recombinant erythropoietin is much more meaningful than Kt/V, URR or any measure of dialysis dose.

Erythropoietin Response to Anemia

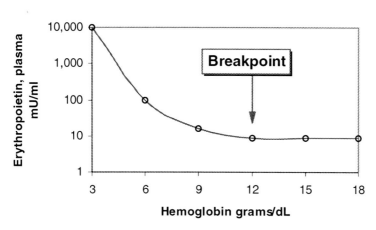

Figure 35 - Erythropoietin response

Contraindications

Most dialysis patients receive epoetin. *Reported* side effects are rare. The original studies of Eschbach and Adamson[19] reported patients with increased hypertension and increased serum potassium within the first ninety (90) days of treatment.

Though not reported in the general literature, there are reliable data of individual patients who develop headaches and other non-specific symptoms after IV injection of epoetin alfa. If subcutaneous epoetin is given post-dialysis, some patients may complain of pain at the injection site and develop hematomas from residual heparin effect.

Epoetin therapy is contraindicated in:

1   uncontrolled hypertension either before or after initiating epoetin

2   known sensitivity to mammalian cell-derived products

3   sensitivity to or refusal to use human albumin

4   increasing predialysis potassium to a risk level (K^+ of 6.5 or greater) which is related to epoetin.

Dosage and Administration

The usual starting dose of epoetin therapy ranges from 50 - 150 units per kilogram of dry weight[ii] three times per week. In most cases, the administration of epoetin is as an intravenous bolus, into the venous blood line (post venous drip chamber) at the end of the dialysis treatment. When the Hct reaches the target range (33 - 36%), or the Hct increases more than 4 points in any two (2) week period, the dose is reduced. The doses are individualized for each patient to maintain them within the target range. Dose adjustments are made in increments of 25 units per kilogram. Each patient will show a different response. If the Hct exceeds 35.9%, many facilities hold the dose.

Target Ranges for Hct & Hgb

Figure 35 - on page 81, is a redrawn and *idealized* response curve of plasma levels of erythropoietin in normal subjects with anemia. Note that there is no increased production of erythropoietin as measured by erythropoietin plasma levels until the Hgb falls to less than twelve (12) grams/dL.[1] These data would suggest that the stimulus for a normal increase in erythropoietin production has a "breakpoint" at a Hct of thirty-six (36) if one uses the Hct/Hgb ratio of 1:3 or 12 gms/dL of Hgb. The adjustment of erythropoietin production in the normal is exquisitely sensitive and elegant.

The normal level of erythropoietin in the blood is nine (9) to twenty-six (26) milliunits per milliliter (mU/mL) or units per liter (u/L). Thus, epoetin may be given to ESRD patients in pharmocologic doses. Attempting to emulate the normal and physiologic process of anemia control and maintain all dialysis patients with a Hct of 36.5% is probably all but impossible given the usual, normal, and predictable variations in dose and response to any medication:

1. prescribed in pharmacologically large doses intravenously, three times a week
2. to individuals who lose blood and iron because of dialysis treatment and blood drawings
3. whose physiologic responsiveness to any hormone changes from their pre to post dialysis status

ii. Use dry weight, rather than the pre-dialysis "wet" weight.

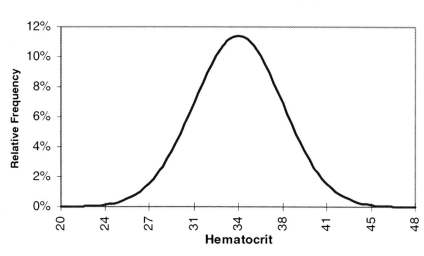

Mean: 34 - StdDev: 3.5

Figure 36 - Hcts for 426 patients

4   who have intermittent surgical procedures, bouts of malnutrition, and take
     multiple medications!

Figure 36 displays Hct data of ESRD dialysis patients transformed into a normal curve. The mean Hct is 34%, the range of Hcts is from the low twenties (20s) to the high forties (40s). These data and analysis of data were compared to data from about forty-thousand (40,000) other dialysis patients. Both data sets reveal a standard deviation of about three and one-half (3.5). Over ninety-nine percent (99.7%) of dialysis patients (and normals) will have Hcts of plus and minus three (±3) standard deviations from the mean.

The range of normal Hcts in adult men and women is 37 - 52%. That yields a blended mean of forty-four and one-half (44.5%). The standard deviation of these Hcts in normal adults is two and one-half (2.5), as shown in Figure 37 "Idealized Normal Hcts" on page 84.

This Hct range in normal adults is far broader than what the American federal agency, Health Care Financing Administration (HCFA) believes dialysis units should achieve for ESRD patients. HCFA's policies for epoetin treatment and sub-

83

Mean: 44.5 - StdDev: 2.5

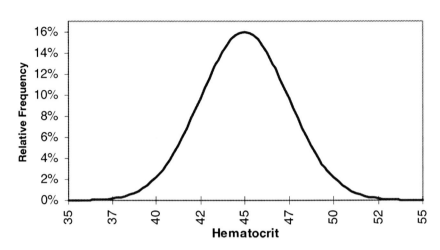

Figure 37 - Idealized Normal Hcts

sequent payment are based on the advice given these Federal civil servant workers by university-based (academic) nephrologists; paid/volunteer consultants to HCFA. We question these physicians' advice to HCFA, the agency that scrutinizes dialysis facilities for quality of care and denies reimbursement for epoetin. If nature allows a normal range and standard deviation, as seen in Figure 37, why not HCFA? If our statistical analysis is correct, it is impossible to satisfy the Procrustean restraint; that all ESRD patients have a maximum Hct of 36.5% – no more and no less.

Hct Target Ranges

Target ranges for Hct are dictated by the different reimbursement regulations for epoetin. Some dialysis facilities maintain their patients Hcts in the target range of 30 - 34%; while others attempt to use a Hct target range of 33 - 36% or maximum Hgb of 12 g/dL. A few facilities will submit special reports to maintain a Hct of 37.5% for a few Medi-Care or private insurance patients. Physician documentation of special illnesses and conditions is necessary to be reimbursed for Hct levels over 36%. In Southern California, facilities who have patients with only California state medical insurance, Medi-Cal, maintain those patients just below a

Hct of 36% or risk either a long wait for or denial of reimbursement. Epoetin alfa contributes about twenty-five (25) percent of the net revenue of public American dialysis companies. It is both the most profitable and the most expensive drug used for ESRD care.

Warnings

Epoetin alfa Mortality

An Amgen® sponsored study of patients with cardiac disease (ischemic heart disease or congestive heart failure (CHF)) was conducted using two randomized patient groups and epoetin alfa. These two (2) groups were maintained at Hcts of $42 \pm 3\%$ or $30 \pm 3\%$. Statistical excess mortality was observed in the patients maintained at the higher Hct range. The incidence for non-fatal myocardial infarctions, vascular access thromboses and all other thrombotic events was also higher in the patients maintained at the higher Hct range[20, 17].

A much more disturbing finding was in a second randomized study of using epoetin alfa. That study showed an increased mortality of non-ESRD patients undergoing coronary bypass surgery. All deaths were associated with thrombotic events[17].

Other Side Effects

IV Versus Subcutaneous Use

Few patients receiving IV epoetin report side effects. Patients on peritoneal dialysis who require injections with subcutaneous epoetin have reported pain at the injection site. The same seems more true for patients on hemodialysis who are given SC epoetin injections post dialysis. These patients may have more problems with pain and SC hematomas at the injection site. If a SC epoetin injection causes a recognizable hematoma, the bioavailability of that epoetin will be minimal. Injection pain may be increased if large bolus doses of heparin are given pre-dialysis (*see* "Half- life of Heparin" on page 97), or if the heparin infusion is continued to the end of dialysis.

Epoetin side effects are:

1   clotted vascular access

2   diarrhea

3   headaches

4   hyperkalemia

5   increasing hypertension

6   nausea and vomiting.

Patient Monitoring

Appropriate patient monitoring is critical with the use of epoetin therapy to avoid complications and to assure its' effectiveness. Nursing areas to monitor are:

1   blood aluminum

2   blood pressure

3   epoetin dose

4   ferritin

5   hct or hgb

6   heparin dose

7   intercurrent infections

8   serum albumin

9   transferrin saturation (TSAT).

Blood Pressure (BP)

Hypertension is a major cause of accelerated vascular disease in ESRD patients. Some have stated that the majority of this hypertension is not due to excess ECV. But, these authors also advocate short dialysis times and minimal dialysis dose (Kt/V or URR). The classic studies by Bower[21] and Guyton[22] on dialysis patients are still valid. With true dietary sodium control, adequate dialysis time, and prudent ultrafiltration, most hypertension is manageable. The remainder of the patients require antihypertensive drugs to control high blood pressure (BP).

Eschbach and Adamson,[19] when epoetin was originally used on ESRD patients, showed that the BP may rise to hypertensive levels during epoetin therapy as the Hct increases. These studies were on patients maintained for months to years on dialysis *without* epoetin. Now, patients are begun on epoetin *almost as soon as they begin chronic dialysis treatment.* How does one separate out the hypertension due to dietary indiscretions, short dialysis times, or epoetin!?

Mean Arterial Pressure (MAP)

To assess a patient's BP for changes, evaluate both the systolic and diastolic pressures and calculate the MAP. It can be difficult to evaluate either the systolic or diastolic pressure alone and assess a trend. Following the patient's mean arterial BP (MAP) is more meaningful and makes it easier in the overall assessment. The formula for calculating the MAP i:

$$MAP = \left(\frac{Systolic\ BP - Diastolic\ BP}{3}\right) + Diastolic\ BP$$

If possible, epoetin therapy should not started until the BP status is known and the BP is under control. Charting the MAPs in patients with severe hypertension on multiple anti-hypertensive drug therapy can be extremely helpful.

Epoetin, Platelet Count, and Heparin Need

It has been suggested that epoetin therapy may require higher heparin doses during the dialysis treatment. It is advisable to monitor clotting studies during the initiation phase of epoetin therapy to establish any changes necessary in heparin therapy during the dialysis treatment. There are reports of an increase in clotting of dialyzers during dialysis with initiation of epoetin therapy. Small increases in heparin were reported to alleviate this problem. In some cases there has been an increase in the clotting of the patient's access. Small dose aspirin therapy may resolve this problem. Epoetin is a growth factor for not only for RBC manufacture, but also for platelet production[23]. The increased reported clotting with *initiation* of epoetin therapy probably has little to do with the increase in the patient's Hct, but everything to do with vessel stenosis, heparinization, and the *increased platelet count* which is common with epoetin therapy.

Blood Chemistries

An increase in appetite and food intake occurs with epoetin therapy and an increased Hct. This leads to increases in pre-dialysis potassium, BUN, serum creatinine, and phosphate levels. Dietary counseling is critical, especially to avoid hyperkalemia. It is important to stress the need for compliance with the renal diet in all patients on epoetin therapy. The pre-dialysis serum creatinine will increase as skeletal muscle increases.

Hemodialysis Prescription

As the Hct increases, the percentage of plasma volume decreases. With the decrease in plasma volume, dialysis becomes less efficient. In conjunction with an increase in dietary intake, less efficient dialysis therapy accounts –in part– for the rise in pre-dialysis blood chemistry values (BUN, phosphate, serum creatinine and potassium). It is necessary to adjust dialysis prescriptions to compensate for these changes. Dialysis treatment changes should include an increase in treatment time, an increase in blood flow rates, and a change to a high performance dialyzer.

Benefits of Epoetin Therapy

The general benefits of epoetin therapy are outstanding. There is an overall improvement in the quality of life for patients showing an increase in Hct levels. Benefits include an increase in appetite, increase in sense of well-being, increase in activity and energy levels, and a decrease in the need for transfusions. Very recent studies suggest that higher Hcts reduce the incidence of hospitalizations (all other factors being equal) and lower mortality rates.

The ESRD Patient with a High Hct

There are no published data on dialysis patients with sustained Hcts over 40% who were formally epoetin therapy dependent. The Amgen® study on evaluating high hematocrits was terminated because they believed the preliminary data showed (statistically) that Hcts greater than 42% ± 3% were associated with an increase in mortality[20,17].

If an average size patient (70 Kg) is ultrafiltered four (4) kilograms during dialysis, the Hct can expect to increase about 6 to 8 points. If that patient has a Hct pre-dialysis of 48%, this patient will have a post Hct that is known to be associated with increased risk of vascular thrombotic events in *normal individuals*. High Hcts have been reported as being associated with an increased risk of thrombosis of arteriovenous fistulae.

With the advent of epoetin therapy, some nephrologists expressed concerns regarding the potential risks to the patients with high Hcts. A major concern was diastolic hypertension due to the increase in:

1 RBC mass

2 increased blood viscosity

3 increased peripheral vascular resistance

4 increased arteriolar resistance.

An increase in blood viscosity may cause: myocardial or other organ infarcts, a decrease in dialyzer clearance, and uncontrollable hypertension. These are still valid issues. High Hcts in dialysis patients may become a serious side-effect as it is in dialysis patients who have had a successful renal transplant.

Erythrocytosis

Some ten to twenty (10 - 20) percent of patients who receive a successful renal transplantation develop high Hcts. If the Hct remains over 50%, these patients require treatment by phebotomy or drugs to inhibit RBC production or erythropoietin. The renal transplant literature speaks of this condition as erythrocytosis and defines it as a treatable condition when the Hct is 50% or greater.

True Erythrocytosis

True erythrocytosis is an increase in the total RBC mass, with normal or near normal plasma volume and is due to some secondary –non hematologic disorder– or disease.

Relative Erythrocytosis

Not all patients who have Hcts over 50% have true erythrocytosis. Some have relative erythrocytosis with a near normal RBC mass, an elevated Hct, and thus a contracted plasma volume. This is akin to the state of a dialysis patient post dialysis after vigorous ultrafiltration.

A medical condition called stress polycythemia is also associated with a contraction of the plasma volume in executive type individuals. This may be due to their sensitivity to borderline elevated corticosteroid levels caused by their life style. True erythrocytosis is not a primary bone marrow disease and may be related to one of the transplant drugs used to suppress rejection. Erythrocytosis is a serious problem in some post renal transplant patients.

As the number of dialysis patients achieve independence from epoetin therapy, and their Hcts continue to increase, we believe that relative and true erythocytosis may surface as serious issues. It should also be remembered that epoetin is made from cultured cells, it is recombinant, and the solution it is derived from must be treated to remove contaminants. Erythrocytosis in renal transplant patients was described before epoetin was available.

Patients post renal transplantation may have erythropoietin levels greater than normal which will respond to drugs, such as theophylline, which inhibit erythropoietin synthesis. Thrombotic events have occurred in these otherwise successful renal transplant patients.

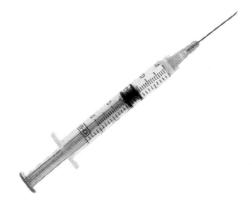

Anticoagulation Therapy

Early in their training, medical and nursing students learn to draw venous blood from normal volunteers using a dry syringe connected to a dry steel needle.

For some, both student and volunteer, this is a traumatic event. If multiple needle sticks are performed before the vein is successfully entered, the blood rapidly clots in the needle and syringe. Even with a clean and deft placement of the needle, blood begins to clot as soon as it strikes a foreign surface. To ensure that any blood test that requires whole blood be accurate, the blood sample must be immediately transferred to a tube containing some form of anticoagulant and quickly

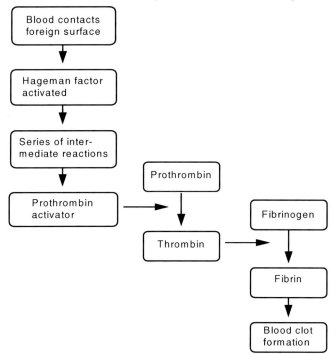

Figure 38 - Clotting Cascade

mixed with that anticoagulant. Normal blood clots in five (5) to ten (10) minutes when removed from its natural environment, the vascular system.

Venipuncture initiates a cascade of clotting events by introduction of a foreign body into the blood stream which both damages the lining (endothelium) of the blood vessel and carries tissue thromboplastin into the blood stream. Clotting can also be activated by any injury to the blood vessel endothelium; such as rupture of an atherosclerotic (fatty) plaque in a coronary artery.

The contact of blood with any foreign surface, such as the extracorporeal circuit of the artificial kidney, its plastics, and other compounds, initiates the same kind of clotting process. Figure 38 Clotting Cascade on page 91, is a simplified diagram of the clotting events initiated by a venipuncture.

Coagulation Factors

Table 9 lists the classic twelve (12) coagulation factors. Roman numerals are used as part of the label for these clotting factors. There is no modern factor VI. These twelve (12) factors, upon activation (usually by contact with a foreign surface) change form, interact, and rapidly cause blood to clot. Not all of these twelve factors are plasma or tissue proteins; factor IV is calcium.

Table 9: Coagulation Factors

Factor	Description
I	Fibrinogen, converts to fibrin by thrombin
II	Prothrombin, converts to thrombin
III	Tissue Thromboplastin
IV	Calcium
V	Proaccelerin, deficiency associated with parahemophilia
VI	
VII	Proconvertin, or Stable Factor
VIII	Antihemophilic factor, deficiency associated with Hemophilia A

Table 9: (Continued)Coagulation Factors

Factor	Description
IX	Plasma Thromboplastin Component, deficiency associated with Hemophilia B or Christmas disease
X	Stuart factor
XI	Plasma Thromboplastin Antecedent, deficiency associated with Hemophilia C
XII	Hageman factor, activated by contact with glass or other foreign surface
XIII	Fibrin Stabilizing factor, acts on fibrin strands to form a stable, insoluble fibrin

A common blood anticoagulant, EDTA, complexes blood calcium to prevent clotting. Other unlisted clotting factors also come into play during the clotting process. There are platelet factors which bear Arabic numerals as part of their labeling. All of these factors are involved in normal blood clotting initiated by puncturing a blood vessel with a needle.

Deficiencies of one or more of the classic twelve factors listed in Table 9 cause bleeding disorders. The earliest described and classic bleeding disorder is "The King's Disease" or Hemophilia A. It is so named because it is genetically sex linked, affecting only males. The converse, a *hypercoagulable* state associated with *an excess* of one of the classic twelve coagulation factors, has not been convincingly demonstrated.

Anticoagulation Therapy

The blood is constantly exposed to foreign surfaces during dialysis. These foreign surfaces include the arterio-venous (AV) fistula needles, blood tubing, and the dialyzer membrane. Over time, as the hemodialysis treatment progresses, the platelets become more adhesive or "sticky."

The blood becomes more likely to clot, *see* Platelet Action on page 94. This graphic displays the major stages, or sequence of events associated with platelet activation and initiation of clot formation on a foreign surface. An effective dialysis treatment is dependent upon preventing a layer of clotted blood from adhering to the dialyzer membrane. Anticoagulants injected into the blood stream at the beginning of dialysis make it possible to perform effective hemodialysis.

Heparin

Heparin is a natural anticoagulant found in mammals. It was initially extracted from liver (Hepar, *Latin*). It is present in liver, lung, mast cells, and intestinal mucosa. The known role of endogenous heparin is to promote fat transfer from blood to fat depots by activation of lipoprotein lipase. Strangely enough, even though heparin is used as the anticoagulant of choice in medicine, it's anticoagulant role in the human body is still largely unknown.

Heparin is the anticoagulant of choice for hemodialysis. It was first successfully used by Doctor Willem J Kolff[24] in 1944 to perform acute hemodialysis. It is easy to administer, has an immediate action, and (in small doses) has a short half-life, it

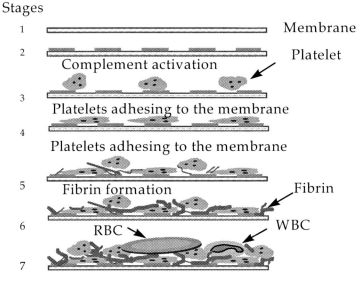

Figure 39 - Platelet Action

is rapidly metabolized and removed from the blood stream. Commercial heparin used for routine anticoagulation is extracted from:

1 the intestinal mucosa of hogs (porcine heparin)
2 the lung tissue of beef (bovine heparin).

The dose of heparin should depend on the patient's lean body weight and pre-dialysis anticoagulation studies. The half-life of heparin may increase with a large IV dose. Good medicine and nursing make it mandatory to consider the individual patient's heparin requirements. Besides the patient's weight, other variables to consider are:

1 length of dialytic treatment
2 dialyzer membrane
3 past history of bleeding difficulties on dialysis
4 blood flow rate
5 recent vascular access surgery
6 recent dental extraction
7 patient's tendency to bleed from small anticoagulant doses; a patient commonly referred to as "a bleeder," with a history of excess bleeding with any trauma or surgery.

Chemistry of Heparin

Heparin has a variable molecular weight, ranging from five to thirty thousand (5,000 - 30,000) daltons. Though it is a mucopolysaccharide and a relatively strong organic acid, it does not affect the body's acid-base status. Heparin is bound to plasma proteins and does not dialyze. The liver is the principal site of inactivation of heparin by use of the enzyme, heparinase.

How Heparin Works

By its self, heparin is not an anticoagulant. In blood, heparin combines with heparin co-factor, Anti-thrombin III. This complex, inhibits the clotting of blood by *directly* interfering with all three stages of the clotting process, *see* Figure 40 "Heparin actions" on page 96. Heparin is metabolized, principally by the liver. It is not a permanent anticoagulant; it *prolongs* the amount of time it takes for the patient's blood to clot. Even blood in a heparinized glass test tube may eventually clot.

Heparin's *local* effect is immediate upon IV injection. But for full systemic anti-coagulation, the heparin must circulate from its injection point to the heart, out through the arterial circulation, and back to the right atrium of the heart more than once for full mixing. It takes about three to five minutes for full systemic heparin-ization.

How Heparin Is Supplied

Heparin is a sterile solution, dispensed from multiple dose vials for intravenous injection. The usual concentration for hemodialysis is 1000 USP units per millili-ter (1000 u/mL). It is also available in concentrations of 5,000 u/mL and 10,000 u/mL. A 1999 estimate in Southern California found that from one-third (1/3) to forty percent (40%) of dialysis units use single, bolus injection of heparin. This form of heparinization is associated with lower supply costs. The latter two (2) concentrations of heparin noted above may exist in these dialysis facilities so that small, less expensive syringes, may be used to give a large IV bolus dose of hep-

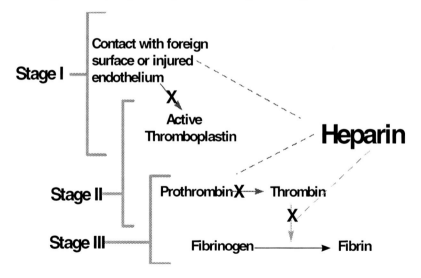

Figure 40 - Heparin actions

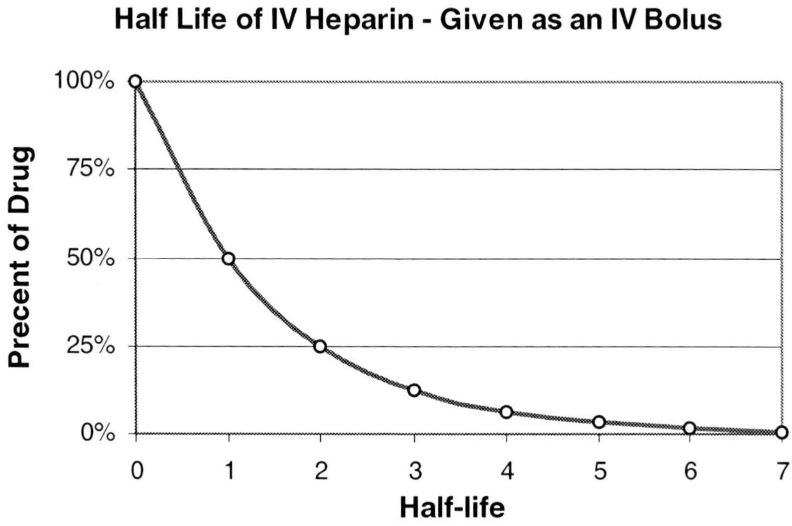

Half Life of IV Heparin - Given as an IV Bolus

Figure 41 - Half- life of Heparin

arin. ***Read all drug labels carefully, especially heparin vials,*** to make certain you are using the correct concentration.

Heparin Half-Life

In healthy adults, the plasma half-life of heparin varies from thirty to ninety (30 - 90) minutes. One study showed the half-life in dialysis patients, varied from twenty-nine to one-hundred and fourteen (29 -114) minutes[25]. The *half-life* of a biologic substance is the amount of time the body takes to metabolize, excrete, or inactivate half the amount of the initial concentration. It takes seven (7) half-lives to remove over ninety-nine percent (99.2%) of a single IV heparin injection. It is an unhappy fact that in Southern California, principally to decrease supply costs, many dialysis units give a single large bolus of IV heparin from 8,000 to 20,000 units. Large doses increase the half-life of heparin.

TJ McAvoy[26] studied the half-life (t½) of heparin in normal volunteers, using bolus injections of heparin from 100 to 400 u/kg. With 100 u/kg the t½ was sixty (60) minutes; with 200 u/kg it was ninety (90) minutes; with 400 u/kg the t½ increased to one-hundred and fifty (150) minutes or two and one-half (2.5) hours.

97

Figure 42 on page 98 uses McAvoy's t½ conclusions to display these dramatic changes in duration of action of heparin. This graph indicates that, if the half-life is increased to two and one-half (2½) hours, the patient will have bleeding problems well into the following day. This continued presence of heparin may induce bleeding events unrecognized by the dialysis staff as these patients may appear at emergency rooms with:

1   GI bleeding

2   subcutaneous bleeding around the AV fistula with clotting of the access

3   late, external AV fistula bleeding after the patient is home

4   retinal bleeding in patients with diabetes mellitus

5   intramuscular and scalp hemorrhage

6   exaggerated bleeding post dialysis because of the use of oral anticoagulants such as aspirin or Coumadin™ used for patients with access clotting.

Physicians and the nursing staff who order and administer these enormous heparin doses may fail to correlate these post-dialysis bleeding events with the pre-dialy-

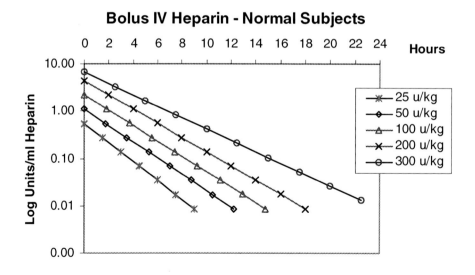

Figure 42 - Heparin levels

sis heparin given. Thus these morbidity events continue unabated and uncorrected; adding to the overall morbidity and mortality.

Heparin Dosage and Metabolism

In normals, IV heparin doses range from 75 - 100 u/Kg of body weight. With normal renal function, up to thirty five percent (35%) of the heparin dose may be excreted by the kidneys. This is just one example of the human kidney's ability to remove high moleular weight substances that are not removed by the artificial kidney. The heparin dose for hemodialysis, –adjusted for no residual renal function– should be 25 u/Kg body weight and calculated using lean body weight.

Estimated lean body weight should be used to calculate the initial heparin dose, the IV push, because heparin's anticoagulant action is limited to plasma. The plasma volume is about 4.5% of lean body weight. Obesity does not increase the plasma volume proportionately. Using an obese patient's weight to calculate initial or sustain heparin dose will cause an over estimation of heparin. In calculating the initial IV heparin dose:

1   use 25 u/kg as the basis to calculate heparin dose

2   estimate the lean body weight

3   be aware that Hct will effect an estimate of heparin dose since heparin is distributed in the plasma; a patient with a Hct of 40% will need *less* heparin than a patient with a Hct of 20%; the patient with a Hct of 40% will have 60% plasma; the patient with a Hct of 20% will have 80% plasma

4   there are few *published* data that show that dialysis patients with pre-dialysis Hct values up to 38% have more access clotting than patients with lower Hct values.

5   estimate the sustain heparin dose as 500 to 1,000 u/hr

6   evaluate the patient post dialysis for bleeding from fistula sites

7   on each dialysis perform a pre-dialysis assessment, a SOAP[i] which includes questions about mouth "blood blisters," changes in vision (if patient is a diabetic), recurrent bleeding from fistula needle sites, skin or muscle bruising, nose bleeds, or other patient specific bleeding problems.

i.   SOAP, a nursing assessment acronym for: Subjective, Objective, Assessment, Plan.

8   evaluate the dialyzer post dialysis for clotting

9   perform a saline flush of the blood lines if blood line pressure gauges suggest clotting of the extracorporeal circuit

10   if the dialyzer is reused, check the before and after fiber bundle volume of the reused dialyzer; it should be the same or within one (1) milliliter

11   many dialysis patients are on aspirin and/or Coumadin, this information must be noted in the patient's Kardex[ii]. If the patient has bleeding problems post dialysis, these drugs may contribute to the bleeding problem

12   rarely, a patient may develop a very low platelet count (50,000 mm^3, μL) from the administration of heparin. This is severe thrombocytopenia. The platelets aggregate (clump together) in the blood vessels and may cause vessel thrombosis!

13   more commonly, up to 25% of dialysis patients may exhibit some substantial fall in platelet counts, if pre and post dialysis platelet counts are measured. these drop in platelet counts during dialysis may partially explain the variability of bleeding and clotting seen during dialysis

14   heparin is a biological product. It is standardized by clotting studies. One batch of heparin will *never* have *exactly* the same anticoagulant effect as another batch

15   because of the ready availability of epoetin alfa, in almost all cases it is better to "clot a kidney than bleed a patient."

Low doses of heparin are sopped up by reticulo-endothelial cells and metabolized. High doses leave more heparin in the blood stream to be excreted by the normal kidney. ESRD patients can not excrete excess heparin, they have no kidney function. Heparin is not dialyzable. The prolonged action of heparin may be far in excess of the values shown in Figure 42, which only depicts heparin removal in individuals with normal renal function. No comparable study has been done in dialysis patients.

The heparin dose should be based on body weight and/or clotting studies with the realization that uremic patients require *less*, not more heparin for anticoagulation.

ii.   Kardex, was a product name. Now it is a generic name, like xerox, for the list of nursing orders and instructions for an individual patient.

Dialysis patients require less heparin because of:

1   Uremic platelet dysfunction

2   Longer half-live of heparin is common

3   No renal function to excrete heparin circulating in the blood

4   The average age of dialysis patients is about sixty-two (62) years; part of the hemostatic process depends on normal tissue turgor and blood vessel elasticity and contractility. These decline with age and malnutrition.

With new patients, it is important –if possible, and legal– to perform baseline clotting studies. Common loading doses of heparin vary from 1000 units to 4000 units. The hourly infusion rate varies from 500 units/hour to 2000 units/hour. The heparin infusion is usually stopped one to one and one-half (1 - 1½) hours prior to the end of dialysis.

Due Diligence For Heparin Orders

Prior to the patient's dialysis treatment, check the doctor's orders and Kardex for:

1   type of heparin ordered (beef or pork)

2   initial heparin push

3   hourly sustaining dose

4   hours of heparin therapy.

If any potential bleeding problems are suspected during the pre-dialysis patient assessment, different heparin protocols may be used:

1   tight or low dose heparin protocol

2   no heparin protocol.

Administration of Heparin

There are different methods in use to administer heparin during dialysis. The most common methods include:

1   loading dose and/or initial push

2   continuous and/or sustaining dose

3   intermittent method.

Loading Dose

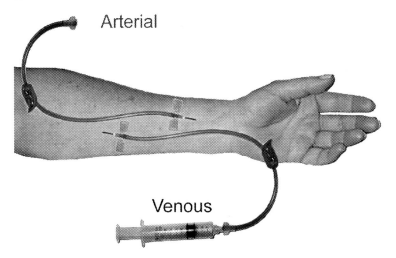

Figure 43 - Loading Dose of Heparin

The loading dose is known, colloquially, as the initial push. This dose is given either prior to or during the initiation of dialysis procedure. It is typically administered *after* both AV fistula needles are in place and functioning. Giving the heparin after the fistula needles have been placed avoids any bleeding problems due to needle placement. If an AV catheter is used to gain access to the circulation, the dose may be administered directly into the venous lumen of that catheter.

Systemic Loading Dose Before Dialysis

With use of AV fistula needles, if the loading dose is given ***before*** the beginning of the treatment, it is commonly called the "systemic loading dose." The initial dose is administered directly into the venous fistula needle (Figure 43), before initiating the dialysis treatment. The advantage of this method is that the patient's blood is thoroughly anticoagulated before it makes contact with the extracorporeal circuit. This reduces the risk of clot formation in the blood circuit. In some instances, this dose may be adequate to maintain anticoagulation therapy for the duration of dialysis.

Heparin Loading Dose at Start of Dialysis

The loading dose may be administered as dialysis is initiated. With this method, it is important that the heparin be injected into the arterial blood line and reach the dialyzer *before* the blood. Clotting problems in the dialyzer cause inefficient dialysis treatments and blood loss to the patient.

Sustaining — Continuous Dose

Policies and procedures vary among different dialysis facilities. The sustaining or continuous dose is delivered during dialysis, usually via a heparin infusion pump providing a continuous infusion of heparin. Some dialysis units do not use a heparin infusion pump and manually inject heparin on a timed basis usually once an hour. With a heparin pump the heparin infusion rate varies from 500u to 2000u per hour.

Doses should be tailored to each individual patient's response to heparin. Hourly doses are dependent upon the results of:

1   prior bleeding or clotting problems on dialysis

2   bleeding and clotting studies, tests, and workup

3   GI or other bleeding problems

4   use of oral anticoagulants

5   physical inspection of the drip chambers, dialyzer, and with reuse, the reusability of the patient's dialyzer.

The goal is to maintain the extracorporeal circuit in a low, heparinized range. If done, the Lee-White clotting time is kept in a range of thirty to sixty (30 - 60) minutes.

Heparin Infusion Pump

The heparin infusion pump, usually located post blood pump, should be standard equipment of the dialysis machinery. It is recommended that the location of the heparin infusion pump be post blood pump and pre-dialyzer, *see* Location of Heparin Pump on page 104. This avoids the possibility of pulling air into the extracorporeal circuit or accidental emptying of the heparin syringe during the treatment. The pressure in the pre-blood pump segment is usually negative, creating a vacuum. It is important that the heparin syringe be properly placed in the heparin infusion pump to avoid positive and negative pressure problems.

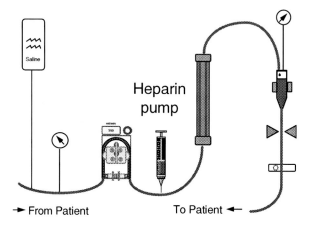

Figure 44 - Location of Heparin Pump

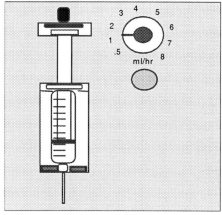

Figure 45 - Heparin Infusion Pump

A heparin syringe is placed in the heparin pump. The heparin pump has a variable speed knob to control the amount of heparin infused per hour, (Figure 45). It is important to make sure that the heparin pump is turned **on** and the hourly infusion rate is set correctly. Hourly charting should document that heparin actually is being infused. More than one dialyzer clotting has been associated with not turning the heparin pump on and not charting the heparin infusion status. Each kind of heparin infusion pump requires a specific syringe. It is essential that the correct syringe size and kind be used in the heparin pump to assure accurate delivery of the heparin.

Each different type of fluid delivery system operates slightly differently. Newer model machines allow the operator to program the hourly infusion rate and the number of hours. Commonly, for patients with AV fistulas, the heparin infusion is discontinued one hour prior to discontinuing the dialysis treatment. This is done to minimize bleeding from the puncture sites after removal of the AV fistula needles post-dialysis. Benchmarks of a properly performed dialysis treatment are minimum blood loss and near normal clotting studies upon patient discharge from the unit. Bleeding from fistula needle sites, after needle removal, should be between five (5) to ten (10) to minutes. Extended bleeding from fistula needle sites causes blood loss and requires adjustment of heparin therapy.

Intermittent Method

The intermittent method of heparin administration is a less satisfactory alternative to a continuous infusion of heparin. Heparin is injected usually once per hour during the treatment. This method has the serious disadvantage of inducing large variations in heparin activity; with the potential for clotting of the extracorporeal circuit. There is the potential for both missed doses or accidental double doses during the treatment leading to dialyzer clotting or extended post-dialysis bleeding in the patient.

Low Dose Heparinization

Low dose heparinization is also called: tight, minimal dose, or reduced dose heparinization.   A low dose of heparin is indicated if a routine heparin dose poses a potential risk. A low dose of heparin is recommended for patients with bleeding problems or risk of internal hemorrhage, such as:

1   immediate postoperative state
2   actively bleeding GI ulcers
3   internal injuries
4   dental or other surgery post-dialysis
5   active bleeding.

When dialyzing a patient on tight heparin therapy the initial dose may vary from 500u to 1000u. The hourly sustaining dose may vary from zero to 500u/hour depending on the clotting studies. It is essential to follow the patient with clotting studies throughout the duration of the treatment to prevent clotting of the extracorporeal circuit.

To check the extracorporeal circuit for clotting, obtain clotting times from the venous blood line. Clotting times should be maintained in the tight range. The tight range is greater than twenty (20) minutes and up to thirty (30) minutes, *see* Clotting Time Studies on page 109. To assess the patients clotting time, obtain blood samples for clotting studies from the arterial blood line. When clotting studies on the extracorporeal circuit fall below the tight range, the risk of clotting the dialyzer and blood lines increases. Partial clotting in the dialyzer decreases the efficiency of dialysis.

Regional Heparinization

Regional heparinization, though conceptually attractive, is so complex and difficult even with the ability to perform activated coagulation time (ACT) tests, has all but disappeared as a technique used in a dialysis facility. It was formerly used to maintain adequate heparinization of the extracorporeal circuit, while maintaining the patient's clotting times in the normal non-heparinized range.

It requires the use of two infusion pumps. Pump #1 (heparin infusion pump) is located in the arterial blood line post blood pump. The heparin infusion pump administers a continuous heparin infusion. The goal is to maintain a desired clotting time of the extracorporeal circuit to prevent clotting. The clotting time for the extracorporeal circuit is maintained in the tight range. Pump #2 is located in the venous blood line post venous drip chamber. It administers a continuous infusion of protamine sulfate. Protamine sulfate neutralizes heparin. The blood is not anticoagulated as it enters the patient. The patients' clotting studies are in the non-heparinized range.

Regional heparinization should only be done by both careful and experienced, trained personnel. It presents problems in maintaining appropriate clotting studies in both the patient and the extracorporeal circuit. Post dialysis, the heparin-protamine complex can dissociate and *heparin rebound* may occur. Heparin rebound causes a state of anticoagulation in the patient for several hours post dialysis, posing a serious risk of bleeding. Protamine sulfate and heparin have different rates of metabolism. Lastly, protamine sulfate –given in sufficient quantities– is an anticoagulant!

Protamine Sulfate

Protamine sulfate, like heparin is obtained as a biologic product. It is of variable potency and purity. Protamine sulfate is derived from certain fish sperm. It is a relatively low molecular weight protein. Protamine sulfate temporarily neutralizes the effects of heparin.

Protamine sulfate is not an innocuous product. Attempting to treat heparin excess with protamine sulfate may only compound bleeding and clotting problems while adding the possibility of a serious allergic reaction. It's use is strongly discouraged.

The package insert included with protamine sulfate will describe the number of units of heparin that is neutralized by 1 mg of protamine. Before using protamine sulfate, review the dosage carefully and obtain a specific physician's order. No dialysis unit should have a standing order for the use of protamine sulfate. Adverse reactions to protamine include hypotension, bradycardia, dyspnea and flushing. Knowledgeable physicians tend to be very cautious when prescribing protamine sulfate; it may clot the patient's vascular access.

Heparin Free Therapy

Heparin free therapy is also known as no heparin therapy. It is usually prescribed for patients with a high risk for bleeding. It has replaced either tight heparin protocols or the use of regional heparinization therapy. Its' name is a misnomer, implying that absolutely no heparin is used.

Heparin free protocols vary widely. Some who state that they use no heparin at all, add heparin to each liter of normal saline solution to prime the extracorporeal circuit. The amount of heparin added ranges from 1000u to 5000u. Typically, if heparin is added to the priming solution, it is rinsed out with saline before initiating the dialysis treatment.

Success of heparin free therapy increases with the use of high blood flow rates, 300 - 400 mL/minute, and periodic normal saline rinses of the extracorporeal circuit throughout the dialysis treatment. Approximately, 100 - 200 mL of normal saline is rinsed through the extracorporeal circuit every fifteen to thirty (15 - 30) minutes, while occluding the blood inlet line (pre saline administration line). The saline coursing through the blood lines and dialyzer clears the blood and provides one the opportunity to view the extracorporeal circuit for signs of clotting. It is essential that all of the normal saline used for rinsing the dialyzer be removed from the patient to avoid volume overload. This is done by adjusting the ultrafiltration rate.

Several institutions administer minute amounts of heparin throughout the dialysis treatment and do not rinse out the heparinized saline prime prior to initiating dialysis, yet still refer to this procedure as heparin free.

Probably the only place where true heparin free dialysis is performed is in the acute hemodialysis setting, especially for patients immediately post liver transplantation or other major organ transplantation. Heparin free dialysis is impractical in the chronic hemodialysis setting. It requires one person's full time attention during the dialysis treatment. Reuse of dialyzers is usually difficult or impossible, due to clotting of fibers when dialyzing a patient without heparin.

Clotting Time Studies

Clotting studies are important to monitor the effects of heparin during the hemodialysis procedure. A sample of the patient's blood is obtained and the amount of time it takes the blood to clot is measured. Common clotting studies are: the modified Lee White clotting time (LWCT), the activated coagulation time (ACT), and the activated partial thromboplastin time (APTT).

Prior to the Clinical Laboratory Improvement Amendment (CLIA) implementation in 1992, the activated coagulation time (ACT) was the most common method used to assess heparin. Clotting results were obtained in less than five minutes.

The ACT is performed with whole blood. The ACT test uses whole blood which is contact activated with a reagent (usually siliceous earth) and results in a greatly shortened whole blood clotting time. ACT's are done manually or with an automated device. Advantages of this method are:

1   requires minimum quantities of blood
2   results in minutes
3   reliable
4   reproducible
5   easy to perform in the dialysis unit

108

6   correlates with blood heparin levels

7   inexpensive.

Table 10 Clotting Time Studies on page 109, lists the different ranges of clotting times and types of heparin administration. Most dialysis patients clotting studies are kept in the range listed as "Normal" in the heading "Heparinization.," The LWCT is kept in the range of thirty to sixty (30 - 60) minutes and the ACT kept in range between one-hundred and seventy to two-hundred and ten (170 - 210) seconds.

Table 10:Clotting Time Studies

Heparinization	Lee-White, minutes	ACT, seconds
No Heparin	5 -12	81 -133
Tight Heparin	20 -30	134 - 170
Normal	30 -60	170 - 210
Extended	60 - 90	210 - 240
Excess heparin	90 - 120	over 240

The LWCT is a simple test. The original Lee White clotting time used three (3) tubes, the modified LWCT uses one (1). The LWCT is not a practical test for a three to four (3 - 4) hour dialysis. The test is labor intensive. The results are less reproducible. If used, initiate all clotting studies with a baseline sample of non-heparinized blood and monitor the patient's response during the treatment. When the patient's response is known, clotting studies are no longer *routinely* required. It is important to document the clotting studies on the patient's chart.

 Note: These are only guidelines. Please refer to these policies and procedures of the dialysis facility for control of heparinization. Individual physicians may determine their own standards.

ACT ≤ 170 sec

1   Increase hourly dose by 500 - 1000u.

2   Recheck clotting time.

3   Maintain clotting studies between 170 sec - 210 sec.

ACT ≥ 210 Sec

1   Decrease hourly dose by 500u - 1000u.

2   Turn-off heparin pump.

3   Maintain clotting studies between 170 sec - 210 sec.

Variables in Heparin Therapy

1   stated label potency may vary +/- 10%

2   longer treatment times increase risk of clotting

3   less risk of clotting with higher blood flows, ie, 300 - 350 mL/min

4   bleeding problems or high risk of internal bleeding and surgical procedures require low dose heparin therapy

5   newer dialyzers are considered more bio-compatible and less likely to clot

6   activity of heparin may be prolonged by: drugs containing aspirin, oral anticoagulants, persantine, indocin, motrin, quinine

7   activity of heparin may be retarded by: fever, infection, digitalis, nicotine, tetracyclines, antihistamines, other drugs

8   brand and kind of heparin will influence anticoagulant activity.

CLIA Regulations

The CLIA regulations were passed in 1992. The intent of these regulations was to reduce the use of carelessly administered laboratory tests in the United States of America. Unfortunately, the CLIA regulations have led to the careless and cavalier use of heparin in dialysis units on a national scale by prohibiting the use of whole blood activated clotting times (WBACT or ACT) for determining heparin activity.

The 1992 CLIA regulations have also proscribed the use of Hcts by dialysis personnel, the use of microscopic examination of blood and urine in teaching hospitals, blood sugar analysis by dip stick, guaiac tests for occult blood and many other simple tests that –in former days– enhanced and expedited patient care. It it a set of regulations that has shackled many health-care workers and physicians interested in teaching. The CLIA regulations have greatly handicapped the ESRD health-care worker in controlling correct heparin usage.

A dialysis facility must be CLIA approved to perform any of the above tests. The medical director nephrologist can not be approved as the supervisor unless he/she has had formal pathology training. Each person must be tested and recertified yearly. These are onerous and expensive regulations. The ACT test is not reimbursable. Nearly all dialysis units are *not* CLIA certified. Heparin clotting studies can not be entered as part of the patient record.

Because of the CLIA Regulations, rather than educate the staff on how to manage each patient's individual heparin needs as was formerly done, dialysis facilities now use standard protocols which lead to haphazard and dangerous use of heparin.

Heparin is the single most dangerous medication routinely used in hemodialysis care; but its use is unmonitored, untested, and unsupervised in many dialysis facilities. We are dismayed by the CLIA Regulations and by the nonchalance displayed by physicians and staff members over the details of proper heparin dosage and administration for the ESRD patient.

Complications of Heparin Therapy

Heparin therapy carries potential high risks to the patient. Staff members should pay scrupulous attention both to delivering the correct heparin prescription and monitoring the patient for any complications. The two most common complications of heparin therapy are administering *too little* or *too much* heparin.

Too Little Heparin

When inadequate amounts of heparin are given, clotting of the dialyzer and blood tubing will occur. The results are loss of blood and a less efficient dialysis treatment. Intra-dialyzer clotting causes a decrease in effective surface area of the dialyzer. The loss of surface area decreases solute clearance and the fluid removal capability of the dialyzer.

With hollow fiber artificial kidneys, if clotting in the dialyzer is extensive, one of the blood lines may disengage and result in large blood losses. If the extracorporeal circuit clots, the clotted blood in the dialyzer and blood lines is ***never*** returned to the patient.

Signs of Too Little Heparin

1 formation of fibrin rings in the drip chambers
2 increase in venous pressure
3 clotting times below desired level
4 poor dialyzer reuse.

Too Much Heparin

When too much heparin is given, serious bleeding or hemorrhage can occur. This poses both an anemia risk to the patient and an infectious risk to the staff.

Signs of Too Much Heparin

1 bleeding around needles during dialysis
2 bruising and hematomas
3 retinal bleeding in patients with diabetes mellitus
4 intracranial, GI, retroperitoneal, and subdural bleeding
5 pericardial tamponade
6 prolonged bleeding at access sites post dialysis[iii].

Proper Heparinzation Techniques

1 remove all air from blood lines and dialyzer during priming, use recommended amount of normal saline
2 secure all connections to avoid introduction of air
3 assess heparin protocol
4 pre-dialysis systemic bolus preferred
5 continuous heparinization preferred
6 are you discontinuing heparin therapy too soon?
7 if product change, reassess heparin dose
8 avoid stopping the blood pump during dialysis
9 use high blood flow rates

iii. AV fistula puncture sites should clot within 5 to 10 minutes following removal of the needles.

112

10 is the heparin pump on?

11 is the heparin pump infusing at the correct hourly dose rate?

12 patients with Hcts greater than 50% *may* require more heparin

13 evaluate reuse program, good reuse is associated with almost no loss of fiber-bundle volume from one treatment to the next.

Oral Anticoagulants

Oral anticoagulants are most commonly given to ESRD patients that frequently clot their AV fistula or other blood access. Acute or chronic phlebitis, coronary artery disease, transient ischemic attacks (TIAs), and vascular diseases, may also be indications for the use of oral anticoagulants.

Coumadin™

The most common oral anticoagulant is Coumadin. Coumadin delays coagulation by interfering with vitamin K's action in the manufacture of prothombin. Unlike heparin, it is an *indirect* anticoagulant. Oral Coumadin takes 48 - 72 hours to have its full effect on prothrombin production. Managing the dose of Coumadin requires that the physician first determine the patient's prothombin time (PT) then order an initial loading dose. By evaluating the patient's subsequent daily PT, a maintenance Coumadin dose is determined. Maintenance dose adjustments are made by using the results of the PT. Never draw a PT after heparin has been given as it will prolong the PT!

Patient education is essential for oral anticoagulant therapy to be successful. The patient should report any unusual bleeding tendencies such as: bruising; petechiae (small, purplish spots on skin); bleeding from the mouth, nose, rectum and ears; blood in stools or urine; and prolonged oozing of blood from minor cuts or abrasions.

Prothombin Time

The PT is the test used to monitor Coumadin therapy. The results of this test are expressed in time, in seconds. The control values for PT vary from eleven to thirteen (11 - 13) seconds and reflect the PT found in normal individuals.

If a person has a deficiency of a clotting factor in the extrinsic clotting pathway, (*see* Three stages of Clotting on page 37), or is on Coumadin, the PT will be prolonged. In individuals with normal clotting factors, their PT will be the same or very close to the control PT.

Patients on Coumadin can have normal, near normal, or substantial prolongation of the PT. For example, if the patient's PT is twenty (20) seconds and the control PT is ten (10) seconds, the PT ratio is two (2). Cautious physicians dealing with ESRD patient's who clot their vascular access frequently, may select therapeutic PT values of one to three (1 - 3) seconds greater than the control PT. Both PT values, control and patient's, must be reported as the control PT is not constant.

International Normalized Ratio (INR)

The PT test uses tissue thromboplastin as a reagent to perform the clotting test. This thromboplastin is extracted from brain tissue. The potency of thomboplastin varies, because it is a biologic product. Human brain thromboplastin is used in Europe and rabbit thromboplastin is used in the USA to perform PT tests. The WHO, in cooperation with other international agencies, developed a WHO reference thromboplastin. The INR is that PT ratio that would be obtained if the WHO reference thromboplastin was used for the test. Many USA laboratories that perform PTs now report PT tests as an INR. In order to do so, these laboratories apply an International sensitivity index (ISI) to calculate the INR. The formula for the INR is:

$$INR = \left(\frac{Patient's\ PT}{Mean\ of\ PT\ normal\ range}\right)^{ISI}$$

The INR is the ratio of the patient's PT divided by the control (mean of the normal PT range) *raised to the power* of the ISI. The ISI varies with different thromboplastins. Figure 46, on page 115 was plotted using an ISI of 2.08 and displays the relationship between the PT ratio and the INR. The INR is *not* the same as the ratio of the patient's PT divided by the control PT. In Figure 46, note that the only point where the PT ratio and the INR are the same is at the value of one (1). If the patient's PT is twenty-two seconds (22) and the control is ten (10) seconds, the PT ratio is two (2.2). The INR for that PT ratio is about five (5.1); because the PT ratio is raised to the power of the ISI. An INR of about 1.5 is used for ESRD patients placed on Coumadin to prevent vascular access clotting.

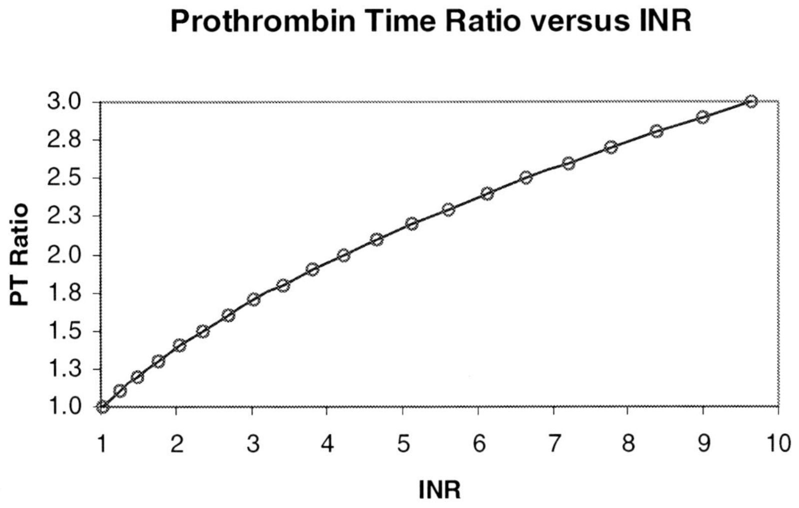

Prothrombin Time Ratio versus INR

Figure 46 - PT Ratio versus INR

Aspirin

Aspirin decreases platelet adhesiveness (stickiness) and increases the hematologic test which measures a defect in normal skin bleeding (bleeding time). Given with Coumadin, there is at least one report that the risk of bleeding is increased when both drugs are given simultaneously. Uremic patients demonstrate platelet factor defects, including a platelet factor 3 defect. Aspirin's action on inhibiting platelet aggregation and functioning is different and *may be additive* to this uremic platelet dysfunction.

A single dose of aspirin in normal individuals may causing measurable bleeding problems for five (5) or more days. This is true probably because the normal platelet's life-span is seven to ten (7 - 10) days. By the fifth (5th) day after a single dose of aspirin, at least fifty percent (50%) of the platelets effected by aspirin have been replaced by normal platelets. In normals, bleeding complications are greater when there is an additional cause for bleeding such as childbirth. Increased post-partum bleeding after aspirin has been reported in both mother and infant. One

115

can safely assume that a hemodialysis treatment adds an additional bleeding risk for patients taking aspirin.

Occasionally, aspirin is ordered in smaller than usual doses for patients who consistently clot their accesses. Aspirin has a direct erosive effect on the stomach lining, the gastric mucosa. This direct chemical effect can cause GI bleeding in normal individuals. Often aspirin is combined with an antacid to minimize its effect on the GI tract to help prevent gastric irritation and bleeding.

The only simple –semi-reliable– blood test used to verify that a patient is taking aspirin is an increase in that patient's bleeding time (based on a bleeding time prior to starting aspirin therapy). Knowledge about the patient's daily dosage of aspirin is not as demanding as Coumadin as there is no test such as the PT to test for aspirin's effects on blood clotting and platelet adhesiveness. It is very important that the dialysis staff know if the patient is taking one or both of these common oral anticoagulants.

Knowledge about the dialysis patient's oral anticoagulant regiment is an important assessment in determining heparin need and in assessing excessive post-dialysis bleeding.

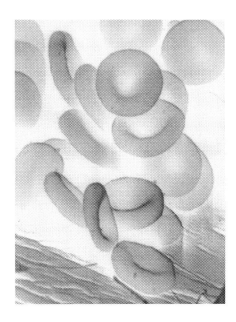

Glossary of Terms

Caveat Lector

The following is a glossary of words and phrases used in this monograph. If there is a synonym for the word to be defined; that synonym may the only definition used.... Most definitions are brief. Sometimes, information is added to perk the long term memory of the reader. Less brief definitions may occur for words that are of particular importance in ESRD.

These definitions are unlike those in Dorland's and Stedman's medical dictionaries. Those authorities may mystify students with their medical completeness and complexity. These brief definitions apply to ESRD patients. These definitions do not fully describe or define:

- normal physiology
- acute renal failure states
- other pathophysiologic states.

Word(s)	Definition
AAMI	Association for the Advancement of Medical Instrumentation. AAMI makes recommendations as to water treatment standards, they have no authority or ability to enforce standards.
Acetic acid	Distilled white vinegar, five percent (5%) acetic acid, is commonly used in hemodialysis machinery. It is used to remove a precipitate from the fluid path of the dialysis machine caused by bicarbonate containing dialysate.

Word(s)	Definition
Acronym	A word formed from the initial letters of a name, such as "TWAIN" for "**T**echnology **W**ithout **A**n **I**nteresting **N**ame," or by combining initial letters or parts of a series of words, such as RADAR for: **RA**dio **D**etecting **A**nd **R**anging.
Acute phase reactant	A group of diverse proteins that seem to be involved in the response to inflammation, infection, disease, malnutrition, and other illnesses. Important in ESRD as ferritin and transferrin are acute phase reactants.
Adhesiveness	Stickiness.
Air embolism	Obstruction of a blood flow in a blood vessel by air.
AK	The acronym for an artificial kidney. See "Dialyzer."
Albumin	A major plasma protein. Present in both plasma and serum, usually measured as serum albumin from clotted blood. A normal serum albumin aids in preventing edema. The serum albumin is the simplest measure to assess the nutritional status of the ESRD patient.
Aldosterone	A hormone secreted by cells in the kidney. May be secreted when the body senses (sometimes incorrectly) that too much sodium has been lost (such as in sweating) which results in a low blood volume. May lead to edema formation in patients with heart disease. Causes sodium to be retained and potassium to be excreted by the kidney.

118

Word(s)	Definition
Alfa	Used as a substitute for the Greek letter "alpha" in a chemical compound's name. A term used by the United States Adopted Names (USAN) committee which substituted the letter "f" for "ph" to promote clarity. See USAN.
Allergic reaction	A group of signs and symptoms: hives, sneezing, wheezing, itching skin or nose, et cetera due to the body's defense reactions to a foreign protein or other allergen. Eg: the signs and symptoms of hay-fever comprise that of an allergic reaction to pollens in the air.
ALT	Alanine aminotransferase. An enzyme released into the blood with liver injury; same as the SGPT test.
Aluminum toxicity	A disease state associated with high blood and bone marrow Aluminum. Occurs with improperly treated water used to make dialysate and/or long term ingestion of aluminum containing antacids. Causes bone disease in dialysis patients, aluminum related osteomalacia and is associated with a resistant microcytic anemia.
America	Commonly used by the inhabitants of the United States of America (USA) and its protectorates to mean themselves (Americans) and their location. Actually applies to all who live in North and South America.
Amino acid	A small organic compound containing both an amino group (NH_2) and an organic acid group (COOH). A building block used to make proteins.

Word(s)	Definition
Amylase	A starch splitting enzyme found in: saliva, blood, and pancreatic secretions. May be elevated with injury to the pancreas.
Anaphylactic Reaction	Classically described as occurring only after being previously being exposed to the allergen that causes the reaction. Initiated by the combination of the antigen with an antibody. An immediate kind of immunologic (allergic) reaction with contraction of smooth muscle (wheezing, Shortness of Breath (SOB)) and dilation of capillaries (flushing, rash, shock).
Anastomosis	Commonly a connection of two (2) vessels such as an artery and vein to form an A-V fistula. In a Cimino or native fistula, the anastomosis is located under the surgical scar, usually near the wrist if in the lower arm.
Anemia	The clinical state of less than a normal number of RBCs. Anemias are classified by the size of the RBC: normocytic, microcytic, or macrocytic. The anemia of uremia, without iron deficiency, is normocytic.
Anemia, causes of	In the ESRD patient, the main causes of anemia are: a decrease in the production of the hormone erythropoietin, malnutrition, and iron deficiency. Additional causes include shortened red cell survival, hemolysis, uremic toxins, blood loss from dialysis therapy, folate deficiency, aluminum toxicity, osteitis fibrosa cystica and transfusion suppression.
Aneurysm	Localized abnormal dilatation of a blood vessel.

120

Word(s)	Definition
Antibody	A protein substance produced in the blood or tissues in response to a specific antigen, such as a bacterium or a toxin. Antibodies may destroy or weaken the antigen or serve as a marker of a recent or past infection.
Anticoagulant	"Anti = against" "coagulation = clotting". A drug or substance that will block or suppress the clotting of blood.
Antidiuretic Hormone (ADH)	ADH is secreted from the posterior portion of the pituitary gland in the brain as in response to changes in solute concentration in body fluids. Causes the distal tubules in the kidney to be more permeable to water. More water is reabsorbed into blood and less urine secreted. In patients with normal renal function, may lead to a low serum sodium from "Inappropriate ADH Syndrome."
Antigen	A substance introduced into the body that elicits an immune response.
Antihypertensive medications	Medications designed to reduce blood pressure.
Aortic valve	Heart valve that controls blood flow from the left ventricle into the aorta.
Apheresis	A dialysis like procedure which removes one or more cells or proteins from the patient's blood. "Apheresis" means, "taking something away."
Aplastic anemia	A clinical condition associated with bone marrow fibrosis and little or no RBC production.
Arterioles	Small, minute arteries; the distal ends lead to capillaries.

Word(s)	Definition
Arterio-Venous (A-V) Fistula	A fistula is an abnormal connection between two organs. An A-V fistula is surgically created between an artery and vein. Over time the vein dilates and enlarges. A fistula made with native blood vessels is commonly called a "Cimino" fistula, native fistula or simple A-V fistula. A fistula made with synthetic material is commonly called a "graft."
Artery	Blood vessel that carries oxygenated blood under pressure from the heart throughout the body. Muscular, elastic high pressure tubes.
Artificial kidney	Also known as a dialyzer. A device with two compartments, blood and dialysate, separated by a semipermeable membrane. The process of hemodialysis occurs within this device principally as a result of diffusion and ultrafiltration.
Ascorbic acid	Vitamin C. Added to dialysate to neutralize chloramines in feed water used to make the dialysate. Used when normal chloramine removal methods fail or for acute dialysis in a hospital setting. An essential vitamin for ESRD patients, involved in absorption of dietary iron, important in RBC manufacture, essential in maintaining capillary integrity.
Aseptic	Refers to "germ free."
Aseptic technique	A method used in nursing procedures to prevent bacterial contamination of an area.

122

Word(s)	Definition
AST	Aspartate aminotransferase. An enzyme released into the blood with injury to a variety of organs: liver, kidney, heart, gastric mucosa, brain, or muscle. Heart muscle contains the highest concentration of this enzyme. An elevation of this enzyme in the blood is associated with injury to one of the organs listed above. Same as the SGOT test. *See* SGOT.
Atrioventricular Node	A-V node. Situated between the atria and ventricles of the heart, special cardiac fibers that receive electrical impulses from the sinoatrial node (SA node) and transmit them to the ventricles.
Barrier precautions	The use of gloves, protective clothing and protective face wear (face shields, eye goggles and masks) when handling blood and body fluids to prevent skin and mucous membrane exposure.
Basophils	A white blood cell with bluish staining granules that contains histamine and the anticoagulant, heparin. Known to be involved in responses to allergens.
B-cell	Also called a B lymphocyte. A short-lived lymphocyte responsible for the production of immunoglobulins, a precursor of the plasma cell. It does not play a direct role in cell-mediated immunity. See T-cell.
Benchmark	A standard by which something can be measured or judged. Originally from a surveyor's mark made on a stationary object of previously determined position and elevation and used as a reference point. To measure (a rival's product) according to specified standards in order to compare it with and improve one's own product.

Word(s)	Definition
Bicarbonate	Sodium Bicarbonate ($Na^+HCO_3^-$). It is the buffer responsible for correction of acid-base balance during dialysis.
Blood	Complex liquid organ that circulates throughout the cardiovascular system carrying needed components to the tissues of the body.
Blood line	Tubing used to transport blood to and from the patient and the artificial kidney during hemodialysis.
Blood pressure	The pressure, due to the pumping of the heart, within the arterial side of the circulatory system.
Bradycardia	A slow heart rate, less than 60 beats per minute.
Bromcresol green	Laboratory method using a dye of this name to determine the concentration of serum albumin. The average albumin level in dialysis patients utilizing the bromcresol green method is about 3.8 gm/dL, much higher than testing the same blood using bromcresol purple. See bromcresol purple.
Bromcresol purple	Laboratory method using a dye of this name to determine the concentration of serum albumin. The average albumin level in dialysis patients utilizing the bromcresol purple method is about 3.4 gm/dL, much lower than testing the same blood samples with bromcresol green. See bromcresol green.

Word(s)	Definition
Brownian motion	The random movement of microscopically *visible* particles suspended in a liquid or gas, caused by collisions with the *invisible* molecules of the surrounding liquid or gas. Named for its discoverer, Robert Brown, 1773-1858. He was a Scottish botanist investigating the sexual behavior of plants. He noted the irregular movement of pollen grains. Brownian motion underpins the principles of diffusion; the more molecules the more collisions, the more collisions the more movement.
Buffers	Chemical substances that neutralize an excess or deficit of hydrogen ions, preventing changes in the hydrogen ion concentration, *See* "Bicarbonate."
Buffy coat	The upper, lighter, portion of the blood clot; the portion of centrifuged, anticoagulated blood which contains leukocytes and platelets.
BUN	Blood Urea Nitrogen. Blood urea is measured as BUN in the USA. In dialysis patients, the usual range for BUN is 60 to 100 mg/mL. Predialysis low BUN levels may reflect poor protein intake.
Calcitriol	An active form of vitamin D (1,25 di-hydroxy-cholecalciferol). Aids in calcium absorption from the GI tract.
Calcium (Ca^{++})	Most abundant mineral in the body. Functions include: essential in bone and teeth formation, transmission of nerve impulses, neuromuscular excitability, blood coagulation and cell permeability.

Word(s)	Definition
Capillary	Minute blood vessel interposed between arterioles and venules. They contain semipermeable membranes where exchange of necessary substances and fluids occur between blood and tissues.
Cardiac arrest	The heart ceases to beat, it stops.
Cardiovascular	Refers to the heart and blood vessels.
Carnitine	An organic compound containing both an amino group (H_2) and a carboxyl group ($COOH$), thus, by definition an amino acid. An enzyme found in skeletal muscle and liver, involved with fatty acid metabolism.
Catalyst	A catalyst is a substance that accelerates a chemical reaction but is not consumed or changed permanently by the chemical reaction.
Caveat emptor	From the Latin, "let the buyer beware."
Caveat lector	From the Latin, "Let the reader beware."
Centrifuge	A mechanical device used to separate body fluids from their cellular components by spinning them. Commonly used to separate blood cells from plasma by spinning whole blood at a high rate of speed.
Cirrhosis	Inflammation and scarring of the liver.
Clearance	The removal of a virtual (non-real) volume of a substance from blood by the real or artificial kidney. A difficult concept to grasp accurately, as it reflects a volume of blood "cleared" of the measured substance, commonly BUN or creatinine.

Word(s)	Definition
Clot	To coagulate, usually refers to blood. A soft, nonrigid jellylike mass formed when blood clots.
Clotting	The formation of a jellylike substance from blood, if intravascular it may halt blood flow in that vessel.
Clotting process	Complex process initiated by injury to blood vessel lining or blood contact with a foreign surface. Historically defined as occurring in three (3) identifiable stages.
Coagulation	Clotting.
Colloid	Suspension of fine particles which usually adds a haziness or cloudy appearance to the solution. Electrolyte solutions are crystal clear, a tube of serum albumin is an example of a colloidal solution.
Colony count	The number of individual bacteria that have multiplied enough so that each bacteria is now a colony of bacteria originating from a single bacterium. Used to assess the number of bacteria in a blood, urine, or water sample. The number of bacteria counted is often reported as colony forming units (cfu).
Complement	A group of at least twenty (20) different serum proteins involved in immune reactions, collectively called complement.
Complete blood count	CBC, blood tests that measure Hct, Hgb, WBC count and differential.
Compliance	Willingness to follow a prescribed course of treatment.
Concentration gradient	Difference in concentration of a solute between blood and dialyzing fluid.

Word(s)	Definition
Conductivity	Ability to conduct or transmit heat, electricity, or sound. In dialysis, it is the ability of an electrolyte solution to conduct or pass an electric current.
Conductivity meter	Device that measures the total ionic composition of dialysate.
Contagious	A communicable or transmissible disease spread by: "fingers, food, flies, feces, and fomites."
Contaminated	Presence of an infectious agent on the body or inanimate objects.
Countercurrent	Flowing in opposite directions. In a dialyzer, the two fluids (blood and dialysate) should flow in opposite directions for maximum efficiency of solute transfer.
CPR	Cardiopulmonary resuscitation.
Crash cart	Emergency supply cart containing equipment to use in a patient emergency, such as a cardiac arrest.
C-Reactive protein	A non-specific antibody that is used as a broad test or marker of inflammation, cancer, or the presence of a disease. Its name is derived from its ability to precipitate *in vitro* the C polysaccharide present in all types of pneumococci. An acute phase reactant.
Creatine phosphokinase	CPK, an enzyme catalyzing the reaction that forms creatine and ATP, important in muscle contraction. Elevated in plasma following heart and skeletal muscle injury.

Word(s)	Definition
Creatinine	A simple, small compound produced at a fixed rate by the body. The muscle mass of a person determines the amount of creatinine produced per 24 hours. The more muscle the more creatinine is produced. Unlike BUN, It is the ideal endogenous substance to measure both the real and artificial kidney function.
Creatinine clearance	The clinical test to evaluate renal function. Measures the amount of creatinine "cleared" (actually ultrafiltered) by the kidney in a minute and expressed as mL/minute. Approximates the glomerular filtration rate of the kidneys.
Crenation	As applied to RBCs, they shrink and crinkle when exposed to a hypertonic solution, they crenate.
Culture	Commonly, to growing bacteria on a glass dish (Petri plate) which contains special growth media which can inhibit or induce the microorganisms to grow.
Daltons	Unit of measure for the molecular weight of a substance.
Decaliter	Ten liters.
Deciliter (dL)	One-tenth of a liter or 100 mL.
Delta hepatitis	An incomplete virus containing only RNA which when combined with the hepatitis B virus (HBV) becomes a complete virus. Medical oddity, incidence very low, prognosis may be serious.
Deoxyribonucleic acid (DNA)	The nucleic acid that carries the genetic information in the cell and is capable of self-replication and synthesis of RNA.

129

Word(s)	Definition
Dialysate solution	Electrolyte solution that is similar to the normal levels of electrolytes found in blood. Also referred to as dialyzing fluid or dialysate. Flows through the dialysate compartment in the artificial kidney.
Dialysis	Separation of dissolved substances from colloidal particles by diffusion across a semipermeable membrane.
Dialyzer	An artificial kidney. A device with two compartments, blood and dialysate, separated by a semipermeable membrane. Hemodialysis occurs within this device principally as a result of diffusion and ultrafiltration.
Diastolic pressure	The pressure in the large arteries of the vascular system when the heart is filling and the ventricles are relaxed.
Differential count	The percentage of different types of white blood cells in the total white blood cell count.
Diffusion	Movement of a solute from an area of higher solute concentration to an area of lower solute concentration. Can occur when one liquid is pored into another or across a semipermeable membrane.
Disinfection	Destruction of most, not all, bacteria, not complete destruction, usually by a chemical or soap. See "Sterilization."
Dry weight	Weight of a patient with normal total body water and no fluid excess in the interstitial and plasma compartment. A clinical guess of the patient's true and normal Extracellular Fluid Volume.
Dyspnea	Difficulty in breathing, short of breath.

130

Word(s)	Definition
Edema	Increased fluid between cells, an increased amount of interstitial fluid. Edema can be local or general. Local edema occurs with local injury such as a bee sting. In dialysis patients, the presence of edema usually means a general increase in interstitial fluid. This edema is posturally dependent; being present in the hands, face, and sacrum after sleep and shifting more towards the feet with upright posture or walking.
Electrocardiograph	The acronyms are ECG or EKG. An instrument that records the minute electrical currents generated by the heart and displays them on paper or to an electronic device.
Electrolyte	Substance that is able to conduct an electric current. Electrolytes are ions in solution. Common electrolytes include: sodium (Na^+), potassium (K^+), calcium (Ca^{++}), magnesium (Mg^{++}), chloride (Cl^-), bicarbonate ($HCO3^-$), phosphate ($HPO4^-$), and acetate (Ac^-). The unit of measure for electrolytes is milliequivalents per liter (mEq/L).
Endotoxins	In dialysis therapy, bacterial cell wall products from gram negative bacteria, See "Pseudomonas." In general, a substance which when introduced into the patient induces a fever and other foreign body reactions.
Enzyme	Proteins produced by living organisms that function as biochemical catalysts.
Eosinophil	A type of white blood cell associated with allergies.

131

Word(s)	Definition
Epigastrium	Over or above the stomach. The central area just below the rib cage which is associated with the anatomical position of the stomach.
Epoetin	The name for recombinant human erythropoietin. Amgen's epoetin is epoetin alfa or Epogen™.
Epogen® (Epoetin alfa)	The first recombinant human erythropoietin. A genetically engineered hormone that *closely resembles* the human hormone erythropoietin produced by the kidneys. It has a circulating half-life (a "t ½"), after IV injection, of four (4) to thirteen (13) hours.
Erythrocyte	The mature RBC containing the oxygen carrying compound, hemoglobin. RBCs are also known as red corpuscles. RBCs transport oxygen to the cells and carbon dioxide to the lungs for elimination. There are approximately five (5) million RBCs per mm^3 in normal blood. The average life span of RBCs is around 120 days.
Erythropoiesis	The physiologic process by which of RBCs are manufactured by the bone marrow.
Erythropoietin	A hormone produced by the kidney in response to oxygen deficiency in tissues. It acts on the red bone marrow to produce RBCs.
ESRD	End stage renal disease. The acronym "ESRD" implies chronic, progressive, permanent kidney damage.
ESRD values	Special laboratory values that apply to ESRD patients. For example, new ESRD patients may have Hct values that range from twelve to fifty two (12 - 52) percent.

132

Word(s)	Definition
Euvolemic	"Eu" means "normal," normal blood volume, a concept important in determining what is a patient's dry weight, See "Dry weight."
Extracellular fluid	All fluid in the extracellular compartment. In common dialysis parlance, referred to as: "ECV," "salt water," "saline," and "volume."
Extracellular volume (ECV)	The fluids which exist outside the cells. One third (1/3) of the body fluid is outside the cells, two-thirds (2/3s) is intracellular. The extracellular compartment is divided into two (2) additional compartments, the intravascular and interstitial compartments.
FDA	Food and Drug Administration
Ferritin, serum	A blood protein that is a reliable indicator of available iron for erythropoesis. A low ferritin means low body iron stores; one μg/L of ferritin is equivalent to 120 μg/L of storage iron per kilogram of body weight. The normal level for ESRD patients is > 100 μg/L.
Fever	An elevation in body temperature above normal (98.6° F or 37° C).
Fibrinogen	A protein in the blood plasma that is essential for the coagulation of blood and is converted to fibrin by the action of thrombin in the presence of ionized calcium.
Fibrinolysis	The breakdown of fibrin.
Folate deficiency	Results from inadequate intake and/or loss through the dialysis treatment. Drugs, such as Dilantin, may interfere with its action. In pregnant women, folate deficiency can lead to spina bifida or other Neural Tube Defects (NTDs) in the newborn.

Word(s)	Definition
Folic acid (folate)	Pteroylglutamic acids, a member of the vitamin B complex vitamins necessary for the normal production of red blood cells. It is a hemopoietic vitamin present in green plants, fresh fruit, liver, and yeast.
Formaldehyde	A gas, HCHO, which is dissolved in water and used as a disinfectant. Thirty-seven percent (37%) formaldehyde in water is one-hundred percent (100%) formalin. The common error of thinking "one-hundred percent formaldehyde" leads to making formaldehyde solutions that are one-third (1/3) the correct strength. This can result in inadequate disinfection of dialysis equipment and subsequent pyrogen reactions.
Functional	A disorder with no known or any recognizable disease that can explain the signs and symptoms. Common in psychiatry, such as "functional blindness" when the patient can see. Functional iron deficiency means that there is no iron deficiency but the patient is non response to normal doses of epoetin
Globulin	A class of plasma proteins that function as a component of the immune system.
Glomerular filtration rate	The GFR is the volume of ultrafiltrate (per minute) removed from blood passing through the millions of glomeruli of the kidneys. Expressed in mL/minute, See "Creatinine clearance."

Word(s)	Definition
Glomerulus	A bundle of capillaries in the human kidney which exists between two arterioles. Part of a complex, called the nephron. It is the ultrafiltering component of the kidney. The plasma ultrafiltrate leaves the glomerulus to enter the proximal tubule of that nephron unit. There are about one million (1,000,000) nephron units in each normal kidney.
Glossary	A list of difficult or specialized words with their definitions, often placed at the back of a book.
Goal	In health-care, an achievable end. Different than a mission which may never be achieved.
Half-life	Also called "t one-half" ($t\frac{1}{2}$). The amount of time the body takes to remove or inactivate one-half ($\frac{1}{2}$) the initial amount of a: drug, poison, or substance. Kt/V formulas are derived from the simple concept of $t\frac{1}{2}$. It takes seven (7) half-lives to remove almost all of a single dose of a drug. A Kt/V of 1.4 with a three (3) hour dialysis, gives a $t\frac{1}{2}$ of urea of an hour and one-half ($1\frac{1}{2}$) hours.
Hand washing	An essential practice to avoid transmission of blood borne diseases. A sensible healthcare practitioner will wash hands or other skin surfaces in between each patient contact and after removing gloves.
HCFA	Health Care Financing Administration. The Federal agency given authority for paying for medical care for ESRD patients.

Word(s)	Definition
Hematocrit (Hct)	A measurement of the percentage of RBCs in whole blood by:

1   centrifuged (spun)

2   electronic, laboratory analysis.

The spun Hct is a direct measure of Hct. It is usually higher in value than the electronic, laboratory method probably because of trapped plasma. The Hct is calculated from the direct measurements of the RBC count and the MCV.

$$Hct = MCV \times RBC$$

The laboratory analysis of the Hct is felt to be more accurate though it is an indirect measure, See "RBC indices."

Hemodialysis	"hemo" meaning blood and "dialysis" meaning loosening from something else. Hemodialysis is the process of dialysis of blood across a semipermeable membrane to remove toxins, restore acid base balance, and remove excess ECV by ultrafiltration.
Hemofiltration	A treatment that removes large quantities of fluids using dialyzers with high ultrafiltration capabilities. A pure ultrafiltration technique, no diffusion. Usually no dialyzing fluid present.
Hemoglobin (Hgb)	The iron containing pigmented protein of the RBC. Responsible for the transport of oxygen and carbon dioxide. The normal blood hemoglobin concentration is 12 - 16 gm per 100 mL.hemoglobin in grams/1000ml of blood. In the laboratory, Hgb is directly measured, unlike Hct.

136

Word(s)	Definition
Hemoglobinopathies	Group of diseases associated with or caused by the presence of one of several forms of abnormal hemoglobin in the blood.
Hemolysis	Destruction of the RBC with release of hemoglobin into the plasma. In blood lines or in test tubes, hemolysis can occur in blood which is subjected to mechanical trauma or water. Hemolysis occurs in the body as a result of exposure of the blood to mechanical injury, hypotonic solutions, or toxic agents. Long marches of Army recruits will induce RBC hemolysis and "march hemoglobinuria."
Hemolysis, Acute	A sudden destruction of RBCs in the blood. If a tube of blood is centrifuged, the plasma will be pink to red in color, due to released hemoglobin. Factors contributing to acute hemolysis are: copper and chloramine contaminants in the water, hypotonic dialysate, overheated dialysate, and cold sterilants in the dialyzers or fluid delivery systems.
Hemolytic anemia	Anemia that results from hemolysis of the RBCs.
Hemolyze	To produce hemolysis.
Hemoperfusion	Treatment for drug overdose and liver failure. Blood is passed over charcoal or chemically treated resins that binds the toxins. No diffusion, no osmosis, no ultrafiltration.
Hemopoietins	Hormones that make blood.

137

Word(s)	**Definition**
Hemostasis	To decrease or stop blood loss from a blood vessel. Upon injury, most blood vessels will immediately contract to decrease the loss of blood and initiate hemostasis.
Heparin	A powerful anticoagulant that blocks/suppress clotting of blood. It is the drug of choice for dialysis.
Hepatitis	Inflammation of the liver.
Hepatitis B virus (HBV)	Originally called "serum" hepatitis as there was no identifying blood test for this disease. Transmitted by blood contact, also sexually transmitted. Serological marker is the hepatitis B surface antigen (HBsAg). A positive HBsAg test indicates either a present or past infection. A positive HBsAg test, by itself, does not indicate an infectious state, other tests are needed.
Hepatitis C virus (HCV)	Most common and prevalent form of hepatitis in dialysis patients; rare in dialysis staff. Patients may demonstrate waxing and waning elevations in ALT or SGPT for months. The serological marker is Anti-HCV. A positive tests indicates: acute or chronic infection or a false positive.
Histamine	Released from cells as a result of allergy or injury, it is a powerful stimulant of gastric secretion, a constrictor of bronchial smooth muscle and a vasodilator (capillaries and arterioles).
Histidine	An amino acid, essential in infants and uremic patients, non-essential in the normal adult.
Histogram	A bar or relative frequency chart; used to display how different events cluster together.

138

Word(s)	Definition
Hormone	A specialized substance, produced in response to some stimulus, conveyed by the bloodstream to a distant site to stimulate, change, or repress actions of cells.
Human hepatitis B immune globulin	HBIG, a plasma globulin obtained from humans who have a high titer of immune globulin for hepatitis B. Given to by IM injection to non-immune individuals exposed to the hepatitis B virus. Provides only temporary, passive immunization.
Hyperchromia	RBCs cells which contain more than the normal amount of hemoglobin; seen in folic acid and Vitamin B_{12} deficiency anemias.
Hyperkalemia	A serum potassium above normal. In normals, a K^+ greater than 5.5 mEq/L, in ESRD patients, a K^+ greater than 6.5 mEq/L.
Hypernatremia	A high serum sodium, the marker for a water depletion state. Seen in normals when deprived of water in a hot dry climate. Seen with use of hypertonic tube feed in the debilitated patient who can't is unable to state his/her state of thirst. Seen in dialysis patients who are dialyzed with a very high bath sodium.
Hypersplenism	A spleen that is hyperactive in its removal of red and white blood cells. Associated with enlargement of the spleen. Hypersplenism occurs in a small percentage of the dialysis population. Hypersplenism can aggravate hemolysis and shorten RBC survival.
Hypertension	Predialysis upright blood pressure (sitting or standing) of 140/90 or greater.

Word(s)	Definition
Hypertonic solutions	Solution that has a higher osmolality than body fluids. Sodium chloride solutions of 3.0% and 23.4% NaCl are hypertonic solutions.
Hypervolemia	Increased volume of blood. Associated with edema and hypertension in the dialysis patient.
Hypochromia	RBCs which contain a reduced amount of hemoglobin.
Hyponatremia	A low serum sodium, indicates a relative water excess in the body.
Hypoproliferative Anemia	A below normal production of RBCs. The anemia of renal failure is a hypoproliferative anemia.
Hypothyroidism	A physical state due to abnormally low thyroid hormone associated with sub-normal body temperature, metabolism, cognition, et cetera.
Hypotonic solutions	Solution with a lower osmolality than normal blood. A sodium chloride solution of 0.45% NaCl is a hypotonic solution.
Hypovolemia	Decrease volume of blood, associated with poor skin turgor and low blood pressure in the dialysis patient.
Hypoxia	Less than adequate amount of oxygen reaching body tissues. Severe hypoxia results in lactic acidosis which, if untreated, can be fatal.
Immune response	Cellular and humoral reactions provoked by antigens in an effort to remove the antigen from the body.
Incident	Unusual occurrence, requiring documentation

140

Word(s)	Definition
Indicator	A sign of a change, such as a color change on a test strip showing the presence or absence of peracetic acid in dialysate. A flag, a pointer, which identifies something has happened.
Infection	The presence of an organism, usually a bacteria or virus, in the body which causes some kind of obvious or subtle illness.
Infection control	Policies and procedures relating to efforts to reduce spread of infectious organisms. In dialysis, this is accomplished by practicing Universal Precautions or Standard Precautions.
Infectious	Capable of causing an infection, usually by a pathogenic microorganism or agent.
Injury	Damage to some part of the body.
Intercurrent	A second disease or complication which occurs at the same time and may alter the course of the initial disease.
Interferon	A family of glycoproteins with antiviral activity. Given to treat chronic viral hepatitis.
Internal medications	Medications that are administered internally: orally, intravenously, intra-peritoneally, et cetera.
Interstitial	Spaces between cells in body tissues
Interstitial fluid	Fluid between the cells and outside the blood vessels.
Intracellular	Inside the walls of a cell.

Word(s)	Definition
Intracellular compart-ment	A virtual body compartment that consists of all the fluid inside cells. Two thirds of the total body water (TBW) is in cells.
Intravascular com-partment	The body "compartment" that contains the fluid inside the blood vessels. Intravascular fluid. Also, referred to as plasma water.
Intravenous	To give a substance into the venous portion of the vascular system.
Ionized particles	An ionized particle carries a positive (+) or negative (-) charge. When solid NaCl (table salt) dissolves in water, it separates into two ions, Na^+ and Cl-. Ions that carry a positive charge are called cations. Tabby cats that are ionized are not called cations. Ions that carry a negative charge are called anions.
Iron	An essential element needed to manufacture hemoglobin. Developing RBCs require large amounts of available iron.
Iron deficiency	A decrease in available iron and iron stores.
Iron dextran	A popular intravenous iron dextran drug is Infed®. Intravenous iron dextran preparation can rapidly corrects iron deficiency. This method carries the risk of an allergic or anaphylactic reaction.
Isotonic solutions	A solution that has almost the same osmolality as body fluids. Normal saline (0.9% Na^+Cl^-) is an isotonic solution. Normal saline contains 154 mEq/L of sodium and chloride for a total of 308 ionized particles.

142

Word(s)	Definition
Kidney	Kidney bean shaped paired organs located to the right and left of the lumbar spine behind the peritoneal space. Their function is to regulate fluid, electrolyte and acid-base balance and eliminate waste products from blood. The kidneys have been rightly called "God's chemistry set."
KT/V	Formula for assessing urea removal for a dialysis, **not** adequacy of dialysis. K = clearance of the dialyzer, t = time dialyzed, and V = total body water. A simple, formula for Kt/V is: **Natural** Log (Pre-BUN/Post-BUN). $$\frac{Kt}{V} = Log^e\left(\frac{PreBUN}{PostBUN}\right)$$ Kt/V is based on three (3) times a week dialysis. If the desired Kt/V is set at one (1) and the patient dialyzed once a week; that dialysis treatment must have a Kt/V of three (3)!
Lean body weight	An estimate of the lean or "ideal" weight of an adult taken from a table of values which use that patient's: weight, height, age, body habitus, and sex.
Leukocytes	Also spelled "leucocytes." In hematology, white blood cells that have actions against foreign matter or bacteria: neutrophils, eosinophils, basophils, lymphocytes, monocytes are all leukocytes. Though the platelet is a "white blood cell" it is not normally thought of as a leukocyte.
Lipase	A fat splitting enzyme found in: blood, pancreatic secretions, and tissues. May be elevated with injury to the pancreas.

Word(s)	Definition
Liver	Largest gland in the body. Secretes bile for emulsification of fats. Major organ for metabolism of protein, fat and carbohydrates. With the kidney and lung performs almost all of the removal or detoxification of waste products or harmful substances.
Loading dose	Refers to Heparin therapy, given after both fistula needles in place to avoid bleeding. May be administered prior to or during initiating dialysis procedure.
Lymphocyte	A white blood cell with a role in antibody formation.
Lymphoid	Lymphatic system components.
Macrocytic	Macro means "large." Larger than normal RBCs.
Macrophage	A long-lived mononuclear cell widely distributed in the body which is usually actively phagocytic.
Magnesium	An important metal element found in soft tissue, muscles, bones, and in the body fluids. Concentration of magnesium in the dialysis patient's serum is approximately 2.0 to 4.0 mg/dL. Activator in many enzyme systems.
Maintenance	To keep in a condition of good repair or efficiency.
Manometer	Pressure gauge to read blood pressure. May be mercury gravity column or aneroid gauge. Pressure readings are in millimeters of mercury "mm Hg".
Marginated	WBCs that occupy the periphery of a blood vessel. Also means an organ laying along a wall or side of another organ.

144

Word(s)	Definition
Material safety data Sheet	Informative sheets produced by the manufacturers of chemicals and medications indicating chemical information, ingredients, and procedures in case of poisoning.
mcg/dL	Micrograms per deciliter of sample.
MD	Medical Doctor. A person trained in the healing arts and licensed to practice them.
Mean cell hemoglobin	The MCH is the content (weight) of Hgb of the average RBC. It is calculated from the Hgb and the RBC count in picograms: $$MCH(picograms) = \frac{Hgb\left(\frac{grams}{Liter}\right)}{RBC\left(\frac{millions}{\mu L}\right)}$$
Mean cell hemoglobin concentration	The MCHC is the average concentration of Hgb in the volume of packed RBCs, the Hct. It is the least well understood of the three RBC indices: MCV, MCH, and MCHC. $$MCHC = \frac{Hgb\left(\frac{gms}{dL}\right)}{Hct}$$

145

Word(s)	Definition
Mean cell volume (MCV)	The MCV is the average volume of RBCs. It is calculated from the Hct and the RBC count. The value is expressed in cubic micrometers or femtoliters:

$$MCV(femtoliters) = \frac{Hct \times 1000}{RBC\left(\dfrac{millions}{\mu L}\right)}$$

Word(s)	Definition
Measurement	The act or process of measuring to compare results to requirements or standards. A quantitative estimate of performance.
Medical records	In modern medicine, "The care of the medical chart reflects and *is the care of the patient.*" The written documentation of a patient's care.
Medicate	Treat with medicines.
Megakaryocyte	A large cell present in bone marrow, not normally in the circulating blood, that manufactures blood platelets.
mEq/mL	milliequivalent per milliliter.
Metabolic	Refers to chemical and physical changes that occur in the body. Complex biochemical actions that convert food stuffs into energy and waste products.
Methemoglobinemia	A form of acidified hemoglobin caused by drugs which makes the RBCs unable to carry oxygen.
Microcytic	Micro means "small." Smaller than normal RBCs.

Word(s)	Definition
Milliequivalents per liter (mEq/L)	An equivalent is a unit of measure equal in grams to the molecular weight of an ion. A milliequivalent of an ion is 1/1000 of that amount. IV solutions of electrolytes are expressed in milliequivalents/Liter, mEq/L.
Milligrams per deciliter (mg/dL)	Weight of a solute in 100 milliliters of solvent or one-tenth of a liter. The expression milligrams per deciliter is abbreviated as mg/dL.
Milligrams percent (mg%)	Weight of a solute in 100 cubic centimeters (cc or mL) of solvent. This unit of measure is not as specific as milliosmoles per liter (mOsm/L) or milliequivalents per liter (mEq/L). Milligrams percent is abbreviated as mg%. Milligrams per deciliter is the same unit of measure and is abbreviated as mg/dL. It is the more commonly taught measure than "milligrams percent." See "Milligrams per deciliter (mg/dL)."
Millimeters of mercury (mmHg)	Commonly used pressure parameter, usually referring to blood pressure.
Milliosmoles per Liter	Known number of particles (ionized or unionized) in a known volume, mOsm/L.
Mission	The primary and overall purpose of an organization, such as: "Our mission is to improve the life expectancy and quality of care of all patients of the ESRD Program."
Mitral valve	Heart valve that controls blood flow from the left atrium to the left ventricle
Molecular weight	Weight of all atoms in a molecule. Expressed in the unit of measure known as daltons.

147

Word(s)	Definition
Monocytes	A type of white blood cell involved in phagocytosis and immune response.
Morbidity	Disruptive and compounding ill events that a patient has over some time period. For a dialysis patient these include: hospitalization for any reason, vascular access revision or replacement, any surgery, any dialysis mishap, any pyrogen reaction, any untoward event due to dialysis care.
Mortality	The gross mortality rate for the ESRD population. American GMR is much higher than in Europe or Asia. Mortality is the gold standard of adequacy of dialysis. It is most probably related to hours of dialysis per week, blood pressure control, nutrition. Modestly related to Hct, and only minimally related to small molecule dialysis dose aka, Kt/V or URR. A statistical measure of adequacy of dialysis for a ESRD patient population.
Multiple myeloma	A neoplastic disease characterized by the infiltration of bone and bone marrow by myeloma cells forming multiple tumor masses. Usually progressive and generally fatal. Accompanied by anemia, renal failure and high globulin levels in blood.
Myeloid	Bone marrow derived components.
Myocardium	Muscular tissue that makes up walls of the heart.
Nephrolithiasis	A kidney that contains abnormal mineral deposits, usually calcium and other minerals, kidney stones.

Word(s)	Definition
Nephron	Complex functional unit of the kidney. Composed of the glomerulus, the connecting tubule, and blood vessels supplying and surrounding both. Responsible for filtration, reabsorption and secretion of solutes and water.
Nephrotic syndrome	A symptom complex due to a variety of kidney diseases, including diabetes mellitus which produces: severe proteinuria, hypoalbuminemia, generalized edema, lipiduria and hyperlipemia.
Neutrophil	A white blood cell often involved in combating inflammation and infection. The increase in WBC above normal is most often due to an increase in the neutrophil count.
ng/mL	nanograms per milliliter of sample.
Noncompliance	Refusal of patient to adhere to a treatment regime
Non-viral hepatitis	Hepatitis caused by drugs or other toxins.
Normal values, Hct	The normal Hct for males is forty seven percent (47%) plus or minus five (±5) percent. In females, it is forty two percent (42%) plus or minus five (±5) percent.
Normochromic	RBCs with normal amounts of hemoglobin.
Normocytic	Normo means "normal." Normal sized RBCs.
Nosocomial	A new disorder (not the patient's original condition) associated with being treated in a hospital, such as a hospital-acquired infection.
Nutrition	The sum total of the processes involved in the taking in and utilization of food.

149

Word(s)	Definition
Objective	The desired end or goal of a task.
Occult blood test	A chemical test for microscopic loss of blood, especially in feces.
Oral phosphate binders	Oral phosphate binders assist in reducing serum phosphorus levels by making GI phosphate unabsorbable.
Osmolality	Number of particles (ionized or unionized) in a known weight. Milliosmoles per kilogram, mOsm/Kg.
Osmolarity	Number of particles (ionized or unionized) in a known volume. Milliosmoles per liter, mOsm/L.
Osmosis	Osmosis requires two compartments separated by a semipermeable membrane minimally permeable to the solute. If considering solute concentration; it is the movement of water (solvent) across the semipermeable membrane from the side of lower solute concentration to the side of higher solute concentration. Or... if considering water concentration; it the movement of water across a semipermeable membrane from water's higher concentration to water's lower concentration
Osteitis fibrosa cystica	A form of bone disease caused by parathyroid hormone excess. The bone marrow contains fibrous tissue and cysts which replace the RBC producing bone marrow and may inhibit erythropoiesis.
Osteomalacia	Softening of the bones. In children it is due to lack of calcium in the diet.

Word(s)	**Definition**
Osteoporosis	Increased porosity and weakening of bone. More common in physically inactive women of advanced age. A gradual loss of the bone support structure which comprises protein, collagen and calcium causing "dowager's hump."
Pericardium	Thin membrane that surrounds the heart, separating it from surrounding organs.
Peripheral	On the edge, surrounding something more central.
Peritoneum	The lining and surface of the abdominal organs.
Permeability	A quality of a semipermeable membrane that defines how easily of water and solutes through the openings of the dialyzer membrane.
Phagocytosis	The ingestion of bacteria or other foreign bodies by cells such as: macrophages, monocytes, and neutrophils.
Pharmocologic dose	A dose of a drug, chemical, hormone, or neurotransmitter, that is much larger and/or more potent than occurs in natural physiology.
Plan	A specified course of action designed to attain a stated objective.
Plasma	Straw colored, noncellular liquid portion of the blood. Contains clotting factors. Serum is clotted plasma, minus fibrinogen, platelets, other clotting factors, and cells.
Plasma proteins	Albumin, globulins and fibrinogen are the main plasma proteins.

Word(s)	Definition
Platelets	Thrombocytes. Smallest of all blood cells, about 1 - 2 μ. Important in blood clotting. They become sticky when exposed to a damaged vessel wall or foreign surface.
Policy	Statements of problem solving methods that support the stated aims and goals.
Polychromatophilic cell	A cell with multiple staining colors, a young RBC.
Polycythemia	Poly is a prefix that usually means "many." A total number of both WBCs and RBCs above normal; associated with disease states. See "Erythrocytosis."
Polydipsia	Excessive or abnormal thirst, inappropriate to the actual need for fluids or water.
Primum non nocere	Latin for: "First, do no harm." A short phase that, though *not* in the Hippocratic Oath, neatly sums it up. Probably the most important rule in health-care.
Problem	The first thing one must know before one can fix it. Most errors in problem solving relate to not clearly identifying what the problem really is; but go off to solve something that is not the main problem.
Process	A method or series of steps or sets of activities to achieve a goal.
Procrustean	Merciless disregard for individual differences or special circumstances. After Procrustes, a mythical Greek, who stretched or amputated captives to make them all fit his one sized iron bed.

Word(s)	Definition
Productivity	Hard to define if productivity is measured in terms of morbidity and mortality. Usually means how much profit, not how excellent is the patient care.
Protein	Nitrogen containing compounds consisting of strings of amino acids that are vital for all cell manufacture. Some amino acids are essential and must obtained from ingested "animal protein:" meat, fish, eggs, and milk.
Prothrombin time (PT)	A blood test that measures prothrombin. In dialysis units, used to monitor the oral anticoagulant, Coumadin.
Pseudomonas	A common gram negative bacteria. Usually found in water. Frequently responsible for pyrogenic reactions in dialysis.
Psychogenic polydipsia	Excessive fluid consumption resulting from a disorder without demonstrable organic lesion. Synonym: hysterical polydipsia.
Pulmonary valve	Heart valve that controls blood flow from the right ventricle to the pulmonary artery.
Pulse	The tactile beat of the heart commonly felt over the radial artery. The heart rate as felt through an arterial wall.
Purkinje fibers	Cardiac muscle fibers, that play a part in the impulse-conducting network of the heart. Transmits impulses from the atrioventricular node to the ventricles.
Pyrogen	Substance that causes or induces a fever when introduced into the blood stream.

Word(s)	**Definition**
Pyrogen reaction	A constellation of signs and symptoms indicating that a pyrogen has been introduced into the blood stream of a patient. Patients may exhibits fever, shaking chills, hypotension, nausea and vomiting, headaches, and low back pain. In a carefully run dialysis unit, almost all pyrogen reactions are due to patient infections (vascular access infections, ear infections, pneumonia, et cetera) not to pyrogens in dialysate or in the reused dialyzer.
Quality	An intangible measure of healthcare professed by many, delivered by few, and identified not by how short the patient's dialysis is, but how little the morbidity and the mortality are in that dialysis facility.
RBC indices	Originally, the calculation of the RBC size, content, and Hgb using the direct measurement of RBC count, Hgb, and Hct. In laboratories using electronic equipment for blood tests, the direct measurements are of: RBC count, MCV, and Hgb and the Hct is calculated.
Recombinant	Artificially combined (recombined).
Recombivax HB	A hepatitis B vaccine (recombinant), that is genetically engineered from yeast cells. It is derived from Hepatitis B surface antigen (HBsAg) and used to actively immunize against the hepatitis B virus.
Renal	From the Latin word for kidney.
Renal osteodystrophy	Seen in ESRD patients. Bone pathological changes which can include the bone changes of: osteitis fibrosa cystica, osteomalacia, and osteoporosis.

Word(s)	Definition
Renalin®	Formulation of 4.5% peracetic acid, 28% peroxide and 5-6% acetic acid. Functions as a cold disinfectant for use in reprocessing dialyzers. Must have a minimum contact time of eleven (11) hours to be effective.
Reprocessing	A term applied to the cleaning and cold sterilization of artificial kidneys in order to reuse them.
Reticulocytes	A reticulum is a net-like structure. Reticulocytes contain residual RNA which appears as a network of basophilic material. Without anemia, these cells account for about one percent (1%) of the RBCs; with a counting error range from 0.5% to about 1.7%. They represent new cells entering the circulation from the bone marrow and serve as a simple marker for RBC turnover.
Reuse	To use again, especially after salvaging or special treatment or processing.
RN	Registered Nurse. A graduate trained nurse who has passed a state registration examination and has been licensed to practice nursing.
Semipermeable membrane	A membrane which allows small solutes to diffuse across it while preventing larger solutes passage.
Sepsis	Pathogenic state resulting from the presence of microorganisms or their toxins in the blood, different than septicemia which means the actual presence of bacteria in the blood stream.
Septum	A wall, that divides, such as the nasal septum or the septum of the heart that divides the right and left ventricles.

Word(s)	Definition
Seroconversion	Development of antibodies in blood serum as a result of infection or immunization.
Serum	The acellular liquid portion of blood minus clotting factors.
SGOT	Serum glutamic-oxalacetic transaminase. An enzyme present in liver, heart, brain, gastric mucosa, and muscle. Cell injury liberates the enzyme into the blood stream. Highest concentration is in the heart. Used as a screening test for liver, heart, or muscle injury. Same as the AST test. *See* AST.
SGPT	Serum glutamic pyruvic transaminase. An enzyme present in liver, kidney, heart, and muscle. Cell injury liberates the enzyme into the blood stream. The liver contains the highest concentration of this enzyme. Serum elevation of this enzyme is almost specific for liver injury; unlike elevation of the SGOT. A screening test for hepatitis. Same as the ALT test. *See* ALT.
Sharps	Any instrument capable of puncturing the skin. The most common in dialysis is arterio/venous fistula needles.

Word(s)	Definition
Shift to the left	The appearance of an increased percentage of immature neutrophils in the blood stream. These cells have an unsegmented nucleus, they are band neutrophils. In discussing WBC production and maturation, the bone marrow is said to be on the left and the peripheral blood is on the right. In a shift to the left there are more bone marrow type neutrophils in the peripheral blood. An increase in band neutrophils usually indicates acute inflammation or infection, but may mean that the WBC count and differential was drawn during or post-dialysis.
Single-pool equilibration	A mathematical correction for a single pool KT/V. A single pool Kt/V assumes that urea has one transfer rate. Estimates different transfer rates of urea from cells and blood. Little different that the simplest single pool Kt/V.
Sinoatrial node (SA Node)	Specialized cardiac tissue in the right atrium that initiates the rate and rhythm of the heart beat.
Sludged blood	A state of high viscosity blood. Associated with high Hcts or other pathologic states including abnormal plasma globulins. *Severe* plasma volume depletion can cause RBCs to clump together, and possibly cause small blood vessels to clot.
SOAP	A nursing acronym for keeping organized nursing progress notes. Each entry contains: date, number and title of the patient's particular problem; followed by the SOAP headings: Subjective findings, Objective findings, Assessment, Plan of action.

Word(s)	Definition
Sodium (Na$^+$)	Major cation in extracellular fluid. Regulates extracellular volume. Essential for transmission of impulses in nerves and muscles. The level of serum Na$^+$ is clinically used to determine the water balance of the patient.
Solute	Substance that dissolves in a solvent. Sugar is an example of a solute. Table salt (NaCl) dissolves in water to form two ionic solutes, Na$^+$ and Cl$^-$.
Solution	A solution consists of two components, a solute and a solvent. Combining the solute salt with the solvent water yields a solution of salt water.
Solvent	Substance that dissolves a solute. Water is the universal solvent.
Sphygmomanometer	Device to measure blood pressure. Consists of a cuff, compressible rubber bulb and pressure gauge.
Spleen	A small, highly vascular organ that lies against the diaphragm anterior to the left kidney. The spleen removes old RBCs, produces lymphocytes and monocytes in the adult, stores some RBCs, and removes bacteria and particulate matter from the circulation.
Standard	Minimal acceptable level.

Word(s)	Definition
Statistics	A branch of mathematics which combines calculus and probability in an attempt to determine if the collected data have any meaning. Statistics can only suggest cause and effect. A poorly understood and widely used tool. Used to reinforce opinion without having to prove anything. Descriptive statistics deals with simply reporting the size and shape of the data. Inferential statistics uses formulas that involve the interpretation of "chance" or probability.
Stem cell	An unspecialized cell that gives rise to a specific specialized cell, such as a blood cell.
Sterilant	Substance capable of destroying all organisms through contact.
Sterile	Complete absence of any living organism.
Sterilization	To destroy all living organisms on a surface or object. Requires high heat or steam or a gas such as ethylene oxide.
Stethoscope	Instrument to hear auscultate sounds produced by the body. Consists of "y" shaped rubber tubing with two ear pieces and a diaphragm or bell.
Surface area	Refers to the effective surface area of the dialyzer membrane. Measured in square meters (m^2). The surface area of an artificial kidney used for adults may range from 0.8 to greater than 2.5 m^2.
Synonym	A word having the same or nearly the same meaning as another word or other words in a language. In teaching, if one can relate a known word as a synonym to a new word, the new word is more easily remembered.

Word(s)	Definition
Synthesis	To combine separate compounds to form a a new substance or compound.
Systolic pressure	The highest blood pressure achieved during a heart beat.
Tachycardia	Rapid heart rate, greater than 100 beats per minute.
Target	Minimum acceptable result.
T-cell	Also called T lymphocyte. A long-lived lymphocyte that is responsible for cell-mediated immunity. See B-cell.
Transferrin saturation	Commonly abbreviated as "TSAT." A ratio of the percent of transferrin saturated by plasma iron. Transferrin is also known as Total Iron Binding Capacity (TIBC). The formula is: $$TSAT = \frac{Plasma\ Iron}{Transferrin}$$ TSAT should indicate available iron for erythropoiesis. Since the plasma iron value varies diurnally, as much as 30%, and the transferrin decreases with many causes of inflammation; the TSAT is only reliable in healthy ESRD patients. Should be > 20%.
Transferrin, serum	Also called Total Iron Binding Capacity (TIBC). A serum protein that binds and transports iron in the blood. Also, somewhat like serum albumin, an indicator of adequate protein intake. Transferrin is a "negative acute-phase reactant," and decreases with many causes of inflammation and infection.

Word(s)	Definition
Transfusion therapy	An IV infusion of RBCs gives immediate results in treating anemia. Transfusion therapy of RBCs suppresses erythropoiesis.
Transplantation	To transfer tissue or an organ from one body or body part to another.
Trend	To move up, down, or remain the same, with no change. If a dialysis patient's serum albumin is low, its trend is a very strong indicator of survival.
Tricuspid valve	Heart valve that controls blood flow from right atrium to right ventricle.
Tuberculosis	A slow growing bacterial disease of human beings and animals characterized by the formation of tubercles (rounded, nodular lesions) in the lungs and other tissues of the body.
Ultrafiltrate	Fluid that is removed by ultrafiltration. Ultrafiltrate is a very similar in content to plasma water.
Ultrafiltration	Movement of fluid across a semipermeable membrane due to a pressure gradient between the two compartments.
Unionized particles	Non-electrolyte substances that dissolve in a solvent but do not conduct an electric current. Common unionized particles include glucose, urea, creatinine, and uric acid. The unit of measure for non-electrolytes is milligrams percent, (mg%) or milligrams per deciliter (mg/dL).

Word(s)	Definition
Universal precautions	Assume all patients are infectious and use blood and body fluid precautions when handling. Was known as Standard Precautions. Now, called Universal Precautions by the Centers for Disease Control and Prevention.
Upright	Referring to a patient in a standing position, if possible. If a standing position is not possible due to ambulatory status, an upright sitting position is acceptable.
Uremia	"Urine in the blood." An accumulation of waste products in the blood as a result of kidney failure.
URR	Urea reduction ratio. The fraction of urea removed during a dialysis treatment. URR = (predialysis BUN minus the post-dialysis BUN divided by predialysis BUN). A measure of urea removal, not of adequacy of dialysis. Greatly influenced by the technique of post-dialysis blood drawing. See "KT/V." $$URR = \left\{ \frac{PreBUN - PostBUN}{PreBUN} \right\}$$
USAN	United States Adopted Name Council, a committee of representatives from the American Medical Association (AMA), USP, FDA, and the American Pharmaceutical Association (APhA) whose purpose is to devise simple, conflict free, and useful non-proprietary names for drugs[†].

[†]   USAN information from Charles H Barnstein, PhD, Assistant Director, Drug Standards Revision, USP; 12601 Twinbrook Parkway; Rockville, MD 20852, www.usp.org.

Word(s)	Definition
USRDS	Acronym for United States Renal Data System; a federally funded program that collects ESRD data from all patients who are funded through Medi-Care. Eighty percent (80%) or more of all dialysis patients receive Medi-Care funds. The remainder have and care provided by state, private, or Veteran Administration (VA) funds.
Vacutainer™	A type of blood drawing system that uses a rubber-topped tube containing a vacuum. The tube is placed inside a syringe barrel containing two (2) needles, one (1) inside the barrel and one (1) at the syringe tip. With venipuncture, the tube is pressed into the syringe, the rubber stopper is punctured by the needle inside the syringe barrel, and blood flows into the tube.
Vasopressor	An agent or drug that caused blood vessels to narrow inducing a rise in blood pressure.
Vein	Thin walled, low pressure blood vessels that carry blood from the cells back to the heart. Propulsion is aided by arm and leg vein valves and muscle contraction.
Venules	Smaller than veins; slightly larger and continuous with capillaries.
Viral hepatitis	A form of hepatitis caused by a virus. In dialysis patients, it is commonly hepatitis C.
Viscous	Usually applied to an attribute of a fluid, a heavy, gluey quality.

Word(s)	Definition
Vitamin	A dietary essential, necessary for chemical reactions, that the body can not synthesize, but must obtain from foodstuffs. A vitamin is a catalyst.
White blood cell count	Blood test to determine the number of white blood cells per a given volume.
Xenophobic	fearing foreign ideas or people. It can be said that those who use urea removal as the marker for adequacy of dialysis are xenophobic to the idea that adequacy of dialysis comprises much more than Kt/V or URR.
Y connector	Describes the shape of a blood tubing insert or connector to allow two different fluid paths as input and a single tube or path as output.
Zebra	An African horse like animal with either white stripes on a black background or black stripes on a white background; no one knows which definition is correct. Somewhat similar to attempting to describe what is adequate dialysis care. See sections and paragraphs on adequacy of dialysis and urea.

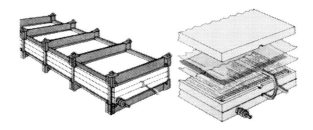

Appendix A – List of Definitions

Appendix B – List of Figures

Appendix C – List of Equations

Appendix D – Table of Tables

Appendix E – References

1   Hillman, RS and Finch CA, Red Cell Manual, Edition 7, 1996.

2   Dierkes J, et al. Response of hyperhomocysteinemia to folic acid supplementation in patients with end-stage renal disease. Clin Nephrol. 1999;51:108-15.

3   Seeff, LB, et al. 45-Year Follow-up of Hepatitis C Virus Infection in Healthy Young Adults. Ann Intern Med. 2000;132;105-111.

4   Bower JD, Berman LB, Remmers R, De Palma, JR et al. What is adequate dialysis? Proc Clin Dial Transplant Forum. 1971;1:61-72.

5   De Palma, JR, et al. "Adequacy" of Hemodialysis. Proc. Eur. Dialy. Trans. Assn., IX: 265-270, 1972.

6   Gral, T. Schroth, P. and De Palma JR. The Effect of Androgens on Erythropoietin (EP) and Anemia of Uremia. Proc. Eur. Dialy. & Trans. Assoc., 7:359-365, 1970.

7   Johnson WJ, Hagge WW, Wagoner RD, Dinapoli RP, Rosevear JW. Effects of urea loading in patients with far-advanced renal failure. Mayo Clin Proc. 1972;47:21-9.

8   Dyck PJ, Johnson WJ, Lambert EH, O'Brien PC, Daube JR, Oviatt KF. Comparison of symptoms, chemistry, and nerve function to assess adequacy of hemodialysis. Neurology. 1979;29:1361-8.

9   Charra B, Calemard E, Ruffet M, et al. Survival as an index of adequacy of dialysis. Kidney Int. 1992;41:1286-91.

10 Sweet SJ, McCarthy S, Steingart R, Callahan T. Hemolytic reactions

mechanically induced by kinked hemodialysis lines. Am J Kidney Dis. 1996;27:262-6.

11   Brockmoller J, et al. The pharmacokinetics and pharmacodynamics of recombinant human erythropoietin in haemodialysis patients. Br J Clin Pharmacol. 1992;34:499-508.

12   Eschbach, JW. Anemia in Chronic Renal Failure, Chapter 71, Comprehensive Clinical Nephrology, editors R J Johnson & J Feehally, ISBN 07234 31175, 2000, pages: 71.1-71.6.

13   Schwenk MH, et al. Potential angiotensin-converting enzyme inhibitor-epoetin alfa interaction in patients receiving chronic hemodialysis. Pharmacotherapy. 1998;18:627-30.

14   Ott SM et al. Bone oxalate in a long-term hemodialysis patient who ingested high doses of vitamin C. Am J Kidney Dis. 1986 Dec;8(6):450-4.

15   Tarng DC, Wei YH, Huang TP, Kuo BI, Yang WC. Intravenous ascorbic acid as an adjuvant therapy for recombinant erythropoietin in hemodialysis patients with hyperferritinemia. Kidney Int. 1999;55:2477-86.

16   Storring PL, Tiplady RJ, Gaines Das RE, et al. Epoetin alfa and beta differ in their erythropoietin isoform compositions and biological properties. Br J Haematol. 1998;100:79-89.

17   Amgen®, Package insert for Epogen® Epoetin alfa for Injection, Issue date 07/26/99, page 9.

18   Kaufman JS, Reda DJ, Fye CL, et al. Subcutaneous compared with intravenous epoetin in patients receiving hemodialysis. Department of Veterans Affairs Cooperative Study Group on Erythropoietin in Hemodialysis Patients. N Engl J Med. 1998;339:578-83.

19   Eschbach JW, Kelly MR, Haley NR, Abels RI, Adamson JW. Treatment

of the anemia of progressive renal failure with recombinant human erythropoietin. N Engl J Med. 1989;321:158-63.

20   Besarab A, et al. The effects of normal as compared with low hematocrit values in patients with cardiac disease who are receiving hemodialysis and epoetin [see comments]. N Engl J Med. 1998;339:584-90.

21   Bower JD, Colemont TG. Circulatory Function During Chronic Hemodialysis. ASAIO Trans. 1969;XV:373-7.

22   Colemont TG, Bower JD, Langford HG, Guyton AC. Regulation of Arterial Pressure in the Anephric State. Circulation. 1970;XLII:509-14.

23   Loo M, Beguin Y. The effect of recombinant human erythropoietin on platelet counts is strongly modulated by the adequacy of iron supply. Blood. 1999;93:3286-93.

24   Kolff WJ. Le rein artificiel: un dialyseur a grande surface. Presse Med. 1944;52:103.

25   Wilhelmsson S, Lins LE. Heparin elimination and hemostasis in hemodialysis. Clin Nephrol. 1984;22:303-6.

26   McAvoy, TJ, Pharmacokinetic modeling of heparin and its clinical implications, J Pharm Biopharm, 1979, 7:331.

Books of Authority

#	Title. Author(s). ISBN. Year.
I	Basic Clinical Pharmacokinetics. Winters, ME. ISBN:0-915486-22-9. 1994.
II	Clinical Diagnosis & Management by Laboratory Methods. Henry, JB. ISBN: 0-7216-2212-7. 1991.
III	Clinical Hematology and Fundamentals of Hemostasis. Harneming, DM. ISBN: 0-8036-0135-2. 1997.

#	Title. Author(s). ISBN. Year.
IV	Comprehensive Clinical Nephrology. Johnson, RJ, Feehally, J. ISBN: 0-7234-31175. 2000.
V	Dorland's Medical Dictionary, ISBN: 0-7216-3154-1. 1998.
VI	Harrison's Principles of Internal Medicine 13th Edition. Isselbacher, KJ, et alle. ISBN: 0-07-032370-4. 1994.
VII	Hematology, Basic Principles and Practice. Hoffman, R, et alle. ISBN: 0-443-08643-5. 1991.
VIII	Hemodialysis Nursing. Pittard, JD. ISBN: 1-892265-00-1. 1997.
IX	Red Cell Manual. Hillman, RS, Finch, CA. ISBN: 0-8036-0145-X. 1996.
X	Replacement of Renal Function by Dialysis. Mahar, J. ISBN: 0-89838-414-1. 1989.
XI	SI Units for Clinical Measurement. Young, DS, Huth, EJ. ISBN: 0-943126-51-7. 1998.
XII	Statistical Methods in Laboratory Medicine. Strike, PW. ISBN: 0-7506-1345-9. 1991.
XIII	Statistics and Probability in Modern Life. Newmark, J. ISBN: 0-03-008367-2. 1988.
XIV	Uremia. Schreiner, GE, Maher, JF. LCCC: 61-10381. 1961.

Appendix F – SI Units

SI Units

"SI Units," is the short-hand phrase for International System of Units, "le Système International d'Unités." SI Units are the modern set of international units of measurement derived from the eighteenth (18th) century French metric system. The USA, deriving its weights and measures from both English and metric systems, remains with a foot in both measuring worlds. American medical terminology and practice uses both English and metric measures. Though the SI unit system is uniform, non-SI units have had to been retained, as shown in Table 14 on page 180. The American symbol for "liter" is "L." The SI Unit Value is $10^{-3} \cdot m^3$. We have included SI unit values where they are no less complex than the present ones used in medical and nursing practice in the USA.

We include the following tables for the reader's introduction to this more uniform and internationally accepted notation for weights and measures and to aid in their reading of this monograph, and more importantly, in deciphering medical and nursing literature that uses SI units exclusively.

Table 11: Seven Base Units of SI

Quantity	Base Unit	SI Symbol
Mass	kilogram	kg
length	meter, metre	m
time	second	s
amount of substance	mole	mol
temperature	kelvin	K
electric current	ampere	A
light intensity	candela	cd

Table 12: SI Prefixes and their Symbols

Factor	Prefix	Symbol
10^{24}	yotta	Y
10^{21}	zetta	Z
10^{18}	exa	E
10^{15}	peta	P
10^{12}	tera	T
10^{9}	giga	G
10^{6}	mega	M
10^{3}	kilo	k
10^{2}	hecto	h
10^{1}	deka	da
10^{0}		
10^{-1}	deci	d
10^{-2}	centi	c
10^{-3}	milli	m
10^{-6}	micro	μ
10^{-9}	nano	n
10^{-12}	pico	p
10^{-15}	femto	f
10^{-18}	atto	a
10^{-21}	zepto	z
10^{-24}	yocto	y

Table 13: Units of Measure

Measure	Symbol	Definition
decaliter	daL	Ten liters.
deciliter	dL, dl	One-tenth (10^{-1}) of a liter.
gram	g, gm	A unit of weight in the metric or centesimal system, the equivalent of 15.43+ grains or 0.03527 avoirdupois ounce.
liter	L, l	A measure of capacity of 1000 cubic centimeters or 1 cubic decimeter; equivalent to 1.05+ quarts (US liquid).
meter	m	The fundamental unit of length in the SI and metric systems, equivalent to 39.37+ inches. Was the length of a bar of platinum and iridium preserved in a vault at the International Bureau of Weights and Measures near Paris. Now, defined in terms of the wavelength of a certain line in the spectrum of krypton.
micro-, micr-	μ	The lower case Greek letter mu (μ), one-millionth (10^{-6}).
microgram	μg	One-millionth (10^{-6}) of a gram.
milliequivalent	mEq, meq	One-thousandth (10^{-3}) of an equivalent; 10^{-3} mole divided by the valence of the element.
milligram	mg	One-thousandth (10^{-3}) of a gram.
milliliter	mL, ml	One-thousandth (10^{-3}) of a liter.
millimole	mmol	One-thousandth (10^{-3}) of a gram-molecule.
nanogram	ng	One-billionth (10^{-9}) of a gram.
picogram	pg	One-trillionth (10^{-12}) of a gram.
unit	U	One.

Quantity	Unit	Symbol	SI Unit Value
time	minute	min	60 s
	hour	h	3,600 s
	day	d	86,400 s
	week	wk	
	month	mo	
	year	y	
volume	liter	L	$10^{-3} \cdot m^3$ or 1 dm^3

Formulas For SI and Traditional Units

Appendix G – "Blood Chemistries" beginning on page 181 displays tables of common laboratory values and the SI conversion factors for these test values. The two (2) formulas below can be used to convert most traditional units to SI units and SI units to traditional units.

SI Units:

$$mmol/L = \frac{mg/dL \times 10}{atomic\ weight}$$

USA Units:

$$mg/dL = \frac{mmol/L \times atomic\ weight}{10}$$

180

Appendix G – Blood Chemistries

Table 15: ESRD‡ Blood Chemistry Values

Substance	Range	Units	CF^i	SI	SI Units
Albumin	3.5 - 5.0	g/dL	10.0	35 - 50	g/L
ALT (SGPT)	0 - 40	U/L	1.0	0 - 40	U/L
Aluminum	< 10	mcg/L			
AST (SGOT)	0 - 37	U/L	1.0	0 - 37	U/L
BUN	60 - 100	mg/dL	0.357	21.4 - 35.7	mmol/L
Ca^{++}	9 - 11	mg/dL	0.25	2.25 - 2.75	mmol/L
$Ca^{++}*PO_4^-$	≤ 70				
Cl^-	95 - 105	mEq/L	1.0	95 - 105	mmol/L
Creatinine (Cr)	5 - 20	mg/dL	88.4	442 - 1768	mmol/L
Ferritin	≥ 100	ng/ml	1.00	≥ 100	mg/L
Glucose	80 - 120	mg/dL	0.05556	4.4 - 6.6	mmol/L
K^+	4.0 - 5.5	mEq/L	1.00	4.0 - 5.5	mmol/L
Kt/V	≥ 1.5				
Mg^{++}	2.0 - 4.0	mg/dL	0.4167		mmol/L
Na^+	138 - 146	mEq/L	1.00	138 - 146	mmol/L
PO_4^-	3.0 - 5.0	mg/dL	0.323	0.97 - 1.62	mmol/L
PTH, intact	10 - 65	pg/ml			
Total CO_2, HCO_3 + $_pCO_2$	22 - 28	mEq/L	1.00	22 - 28	mmol/L
Transferrin Saturation	≥ 20	%			
URR	≥ 70	%			

‡Values will vary according to laboratory and other factors

i. Conversion Factor; the reciprocal (1/mole wt) of the substance. Multiply the value by this number.

Gram Molecular Weight

A mole is one of the seven (7) fundamental units of SI. One mole or one gram-molecular weight is the atomic weight of a substance in grams. One mole of *any* substance contains the same number of: atoms, particles, or molecules. A mole contains $6.02+ \times 10^{23}$ atoms or un-ionized molecules. It is based on the number of atoms in twelve (12) grams of carbon, which has an atomic weight of twelve (12).

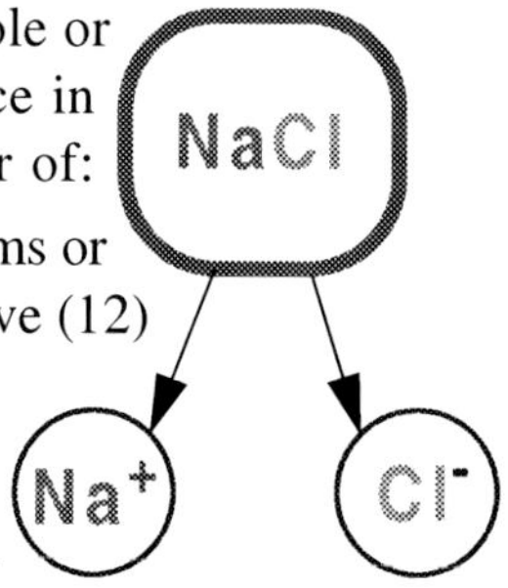

If one weighs out fifty-eight and one-half (58.5) grams of common table salt, that is one (1) mole of table salt; the combined atomic weights of sodium (Na^+) and chloride (Cl^-). If that table salt is then dissolved in water, the salt molecules will dissociate into one mole of Na^+ and one mole of Cl^- ions, (Figure 42). Monovalent electrolytes expressed in milliequivalent per liter (mEq/L), such as K^+ and Na^+, have the same values in mEq/L as mmol/L, (Table 16).

Figure 42 - Ionized Salt

Table 16: Examples of Conversion to SI Units

Substance	Units	At wt	Calculate[†]	CF*	CF*	SI	
Blood Urea[‡]	214 mg/dL	60	214/6.0	1/6.0	0.0167	35.67	mmol/L
BUN	100 mg/dL	28	100/2.8	1/2.8	0.357	35.71	mmol/L
Ca^{++}	9.0 mg/dL	40	9/4.0	1/4.0	0.25	2.25	mmol/L
Ca^{++}	4.5 mEq/L	40	20*4.5/40	1/2	0.5	2.25	mmol/L
Glucose	100 mg/dL	180	100/18.0	1/18.0	0.0556	5.56	mmol/L
K^+	5.5 mEq/L	39	39*5.5/39	1/1	1.0	5.5	mmol/L
Mg^{++}	2.0 mg/dL	24	2/2.4	1/2.4	0.4146	0.833	mmol/L

† To calculate the SI units, divide Units by the atomic weight (At wt), correcting from dL to Liter. Monovalent cations expressed in mEq/L require no correction. See Ca^{++} as an example of a divalent cation expressed in mg/dL and mEq/L.

‡ Blood Urea is used in Europe, note that blood urea is about 2.14 times BUN.

* CF, conversion factor, calculated by dividing one by the atomic weight of the un-ionized particle. First CF column shows the formula, second the resultant CF.

Appendix H – Infection Control

Precautions for Dialysis Units

In 1977, the Centers for Disease Control (CDC) published precautions to prevent transmission of HBV in dialysis centers (Reference B1). In 1987, universal precautions were developed to prevent transmission of all blood-borne pathogens, including HBV and HIV, in health care and other settings (Reference B2). In 1996, an updated system of precautions, termed standard precautions, was published to replace universal precautions for the hospital and most healthcare settings (Reference B3). The infection control measures currently recommended for dialysis units incorporate features of each of these guidelines. These measures are effective against HBV, the most highly transmissible organism in hemodialysis units; therefore, they should also be effective against other viruses (eg., HCV) and bacteria (eg., VRE).

Note that dialysis unit precautions are more stringent than universal or standard precautions. For example, standard precautions require the use of gloves only when touching blood, body fluids, secretions, excretions, or contaminated items. In contrast, dialysis unit precautions require glove use whenever patients or hemodialysis equipment is touched. Standard precautions do not restrict the use of supplies, instruments, and medications to a single patient; dialysis unit precautions specify that none of these be shared between any patients.

Since dialysis patients may, known or unknown to the staff, be infected or colonized with a variety of bacteria and viruses, the following precautions should be used during care of **all dialysis patients at all times**.

Assign each patient a:

1   dialysis chair or bed and machine; and

2   supply tray (tourniquet, antiseptics, if possible blood pressure cuff). Avoid sharing these items.

Do not share clamps, scissors, other non-disposable items unless sterilized or disinfected between patients.

Prepare and distribute medications from a centralized area. Medication carts should not be used. Separate clean and contaminated areas; for example, handling and storage of medications and hand washing should not be done in the same or adjacent area to that where blood samples or used equipment are handled.

Disposable gloves should be worn by staff members for their own protection when handling patients or dialysis equipment and accessories. Gloves should be worn when taking blood pressure, injecting saline or heparin, or touching dialysis machine knobs to adjust flow rates. For the patient's protection, the staff member should use a fresh pair of gloves with each patient to prevent cross-contamination. Gloves also should be used when handling blood specimens. Staff members should wash their hands after each patient contact. Avoid touching surfaces with gloved hands that will subsequently be touched with un-gloved hands before being disinfected.

Staff members may wish to wear protective eyeglasses and masks for procedures in which spurting or spattering of blood may occur, such as cleaning of dialyzers and centrifugation of blood. Face protection is highly recommended.

Staff members should wear gowns, scrub suits, or the equivalent while working in the unit and should change out of this clothing at the end of each day. After each dialysis, (1) change linen; (2) clean and disinfect the dialysis bed/chair and non-disposable equipment (especially control knobs and other surfaces touched by gloved hands).

Crowding patients or overtaxing staff may facilitate cross- transmission. Avoid clutter and allocate adequate space to facilitate cleaning and housekeeping.

Staff members should not smoke, eat, or drink in the dialysis treatment area or in the laboratory. There should be a separate lounge for this purpose. However, all patients may be served meals. The glasses, dishes, and other utensils may be cleaned in the usual manner by the hospital staff. No special care of these items is needed.

References

B1. Centers for Disease Control and Prevention. Control measures for hepatitis in dialysis centers. Viral Hepatitis Investigations and Control Series. November 1977.

B2. Centers for Disease Control and Prevention. Recommendations for prevention of HIV transmission in health-care settings. MMWR 1987;36 (No. 2S):3S-18S.

B3. Garner JS, the Hospital Infection Control Practices Advisory Committee. Guideline for isolation precautions in hospitals. Infect Control Hosp Epidemiol 1996;17:53-80.

B4. Centers for Disease Control and Prevention. Recommendations for preventing the spread of vancomycin resistance. MMWR 1995;44 (No. RR-12):1-13.

B5. Fogel MA. Use of cefazolin in place of vancomycin in hemodialysis patients [Abstract A0992]. J Am Soc Nephrol 1996;7 (No. 9):1446.

Appendix I – Body Mass Index

Table 17: BMI Chart

BMI	16	17	18	19	20	21	22	23	24	25	26	27	28	29	30	31	32	33
Ht	Wt																	
4' 10	77	81	86	91	96	100	105	110	115	120	124	129	134	139	144	148	153	158
4' 11	79	84	89	94	99	104	109	114	119	124	129	134	139	144	149	153	158	163
5' 0	82	87	92	97	102	108	113	118	123	128	133	138	143	148	154	159	164	169
5' 1	85	90	95	101	106	111	116	122	127	132	138	143	148	153	159	164	169	175
5' 2	87	93	98	104	109	115	120	126	131	137	142	148	153	159	164	169	175	180
5' 3	90	96	102	107	113	119	124	130	135	141	147	152	158	164	169	175	181	186
5' 4	93	99	105	111	117	122	128	134	140	146	151	157	163	169	175	181	186	192
5' 5	96	102	108	114	120	126	132	138	144	150	156	162	168	174	180	186	192	198
5' 6	99	105	112	118	124	130	136	142	149	155	161	167	173	180	186	192	198	204
5' 7	102	109	115	121	128	134	140	147	153	160	166	172	179	185	192	198	204	211
5' 8	105	112	118	125	132	138	145	151	158	164	171	178	184	191	197	204	210	217
5' 9	108	115	122	129	135	142	149	156	162	169	176	183	190	196	203	210	217	223
5' 10	111	118	125	132	139	146	153	160	167	174	181	188	195	202	209	216	223	230
5' 11	115	122	129	136	143	151	158	165	172	179	186	194	201	208	215	222	229	237
6' 0	118	125	133	140	147	155	162	170	177	184	192	199	206	214	221	229	236	243
6' 1	121	129	136	144	152	159	167	174	182	189	197	205	212	220	227	235	243	250
6' 2	125	132	140	148	156	164	171	179	187	195	202	210	218	226	234	241	249	257
6' 3	128	136	144	152	160	168	176	184	192	200	208	216	224	232	240	248	256	264
6' 4	131	140	148	156	164	172	181	189	197	205	214	222	230	238	246	255	263	271
6' 5	135	143	152	160	169	177	185	194	202	211	219	228	236	245	253	261	270	278
6' 6	138	147	156	164	173	182	190	199	208	216	225	234	242	251	260	268	277	286
BMI	16	17	18	19	20	21	22	23	24	25	26	27	28	29	30	31	32	33

BMI key:
- Under-weight   16 through 19
- Normal   19 through 24
- Obese   25 through 29
- Morbidly Obese   over 30

Post Test

The following questions are multiple choice. *Select one answer only.* Circle the correct response on the post test answer form located in the back of the book.

1   A drop in the hematocrit may indicate:

    A   Bleeding problems

    B   Increase in salt water retention

    C   An incorrect hematocrit procedure

    D   The patient is not responding to EPO therapy

    E   All of the above

2   Dialysis patients with low iron stores and/or available iron for erythropoiesis will receive intravenous (IV) iron to correct iron deficiency during the dialysis treatment. Identify the most common IV drug in use to correct iron deficiency.

    A   Recombinant human 1,25 Vitamin D

    B   Recombinant human erythropoietin

    C   Iron Dextran

    D   Recombinant human deoxyribonucleic acid

    E   Calcitriol

3   The hematocrit is defined as:

      A   The differential between red blood cells and white blood cells

      B   Total plasma volume

      C   The evaluation of hemolyzed re blood cells

      D   The percentage of red blood cells in the total volume of the blood sample

      E   None of the above

4   Patients on hemodialysis are anemic. This anemia may be related to a shortened survival of RBCs as well as a reduction of RBCs made as compared to normal. One of the following statements regarding the anemia as seen in dialysis patients is *FALSE*, *indicate that statement*.

      A   Intravenous iron is used to correct iron deficiency anemia in hemodialysis patients

      B   Androgen therapy has no effect on improving the anemia in hemodialysis patients

      C   Excessive blood loss through blood sampling or ruptures of dialyzers may decrease the patients Hct substantially

      D   The Hct may vary from 12 to 52% in hemodialysis patients

5   A technological breakthrough in the treatment of anemia via recombinant DNA techniques is currently in use. The substance that is being given as a medication to improve anemia is:

      A   Recombinant human 1,25 Vitamin D

      B   Epoetin

      C   Iron Dextran

      D   Recombinant human deoxynucleic acid

      E   Calcitriol

6   A percentage of dialysis patients do not respond to the administration of epoetin. When this is the situation, a number of factors must be checked. Which one of the following factors listed would **not** be appropriate in assessing the patient's response to this drug?

    A   Adequate nutrition in regards to protein and caloric intake

    B   Adequate intake of folic acid and vitamin therapy

    C   Serum Ferritin level of > 100 ng/L as an indicator of iron stores

    D   Maintenance of BUN between 8 - 20 mg%

    E   A transferrin saturation of > 20% to assess available iron for erythropoiesis

7   There are different types of cells in the blood. Which blood cell plays a role in hemostasis?

    A   Red blood cell

    B   Platelets

    C   White blood cell

    D   Eosinophil

    E   Reticulocyte

8   There are several different types of white blood cells. Identify which one of the following blood cells listed, that is **not** a white blood cell.

    A   Neutrophil

    B   Basophil

    C   Monocyte

    D   Erythrocyte

    E   Lymphocyte

9   When a patient demonstrates a fever in the dialysis unit, a complete blood cell count is ordered. Identify the particular part of this blood test that would demonstrate an increase in response to the presence of an infection or pyrogen?

A   Red cell count

B   White cell count

C   Platelet count

D   Hemoglobin

E   Hematocrit

10   Testosterone is a male hormone which is used on some dialysis patients, primarily to:

A   Decrease the blood pressure

B   Treat infections

C   Increase the hematocrit

D   Prevent impotence

E   Stimulate the patient's appetite

11   The prescribed dosage of an anticoagulant is ideally determined by the patient's?

A   Sedimentation Rate

B   Bleeding Time

C   Capillary Fragility Test

D   Weight and Clotting Time Studies

E   Prothrombin Time

12   The term "anticoagulation" means?

    A   To circulate blood through the extracorporeal circulation

    B   To delay or prevent blood from clotting

    C   To thin the blood

    D   To cause blood to clot

    E   To make platelets more adhesive (sticky)

13   Heparin is supplied for use in a sterile solution for intravenous injection in multiple dose vials. What is the usual concentration of heparin used for hemodialysis?

    A   Heparin 500 u/ml

    B   Heparin 1000 u/ml

    C   Heparin 2000 u/ml

    D   Heparin 5000 u/ml

    E   Heparin 10,000 u/ml

14   The osmolarity of the plasma prevents an excess of fluid within the interstitial spaces. Which one of the following substances exerts an osmotic force to return the extracellular fluid to the blood, which has been ultrafiltered by the blood pressure?

    A   Sodium

    B   Potassium

    C   Bicarbonate

    D   Albumin

    E   Chloride

15   Which one of the following statements regarding heparin is **true**?

       A   Heparin is non-dialyzable

       B   Heparin's effect lasts at least 24 hours

       C   Heparin is dialyzable

       D   Heparin's effects only the last stage of clotting

       E   Heparin has a low molecular weight

16   Signs and symptoms of over-heparinization are:

       A   Bleeding around needle insertion sites

       B   Inability to clot needle sites post-dialysis

       C   Patient complains of continuous bruising

       D   All of the above

       E   None of the above

17   Bacteriocidal compounds are routinely added to municipal water supplies as part of the water treatment process. To prevent hemolysis, these compounds must be removed in dialysis units as part of the water treatment process by using activated carbon tanks. Identify the compounds.

       A   Calcium and magnesium

       B   Chloramines

       C   Nitrates and nitrites

       D   Bacteria and viruses

       E   Sodium chloride compounds

18   Of the following groups listed, which will **ALL** cause hemolysis when exposed to blood?

    A   Bleach, dialysate 96°F, and dialysate 118°F

    B   Dialysate 96°F, dialysate 118°F, and 95 mEq chloride bath

    C   Bleach, dialysate 118° F, and hypotonic dialysate

    D   Dialysate 38°C, 95 mEq chloride bath and 140 mEq sodium bath

    E   Dialysate 36°C, hypotonic dialysate and a OK bath

19   The State of California adds chloramines to the water as part of their water treatment process. Which one of the following methods is sometimes used in the acute setting in a hospital as part of their water treatment system to remove chloramines?

    A   Water softeners

    B   Sediment filters

    C   Reverse osmosis

    D   Addition of ascorbic acid to the dialysate

    E   None of the above

20   Anemic patients show a variety of clinical signs and symptoms. Usually, the degree of symptoms is proportional to the degree of anemia. Which one of the symptoms listed, is not indicative of anemia?

    A   Dyspnea

    B   Angina

    C   Headaches

    D   Loss of appetite

    E   Hypertension

21   When a patient receives too little heparin, multiple problems can occur. Which item listed would **NOT** be a result of this?

    A   Fibrin buildup

    B   Clotted dialyzer

    C   Less effective dialysis

    D   Clot formation in the drip chambers

    E   Prolonged bleeding

22   When taking a blood specimen in dialysis, personnel should wear gloves to:

    A   Prevent contamination of the blood specimen

    B   Protect themselves against staphylococcus bacteria

    C   Keep the procedure as clean as possible

    D   Protect themselves against hepatitis and other contagious diseases

    E   Maintain sterility of the blood

23   The physician orders 3500u initial heparin push and heparin 500u sustaining dose for three hours. What is the total amount of heparin to be given using 1000u/ml heparin over the duration of the dialysis treatment?

    A   Total of 3.5ml

    B   Total of 0.5ml

    C   Total of 4.0ml

    D   Total of 5.0ml

    E   Total of 6.0ml

24   Your patient states that she is going to have access surgery after dialysis
      during your pre-dialysis assessment. In view of this event, which of the
      following actions would be most appropriate?

      A   Wait and see what happens during the dialysis today

      B   Inform the charge nurse, and run the patient on his usual 3000u
           prime and 1500u hourly dose of heparin

      C   Inform the charge nurse, and run the patient on a reduced heparin
           dose, followed with clotting studies, if possible

      D   Give the patient Protamine at the beginning of dialysis

      E   Do nothing

25   The prescribed dosage of the anticoagulant heparin can determined by
      which blood test?

      A   Sedimentation Rate

      B   Bleeding Time

      C   Capillary Fragility Test

      D   Activated Clotting Time

      E   Red Blood Count

26   Improper heparin therapy during dialysis may result in:

      A   Prolonged bleeding from the A/V fistula needle sites

      B   Clotting in the extracorporeal circulation

      C   Blood loss due to clotting

      D   Blood loss due to bleeding

      E   All of the above

27   Which of the following conditions may retard the activity of heparin and necessitate larger doses? Select the ***best*** answer.

    A   Elevated body temperature. aspirin, nicotine, and antihistamines

    B   Elevated body temperature, antihistamines, digitalis, tetracyclines, and nicotine

    C   Nicotine, tetracyclines, subnormal body temperature

    D   Aspirin, nicotine, digitalis

    E   Elevated body temperature only

28   Which one of the following medications prolongs the activity of heparin in a patient?

    A   Protamine sulfate

    B   Folic acid

    C   Aspirin

    D   Deca-Durabolin

    E   None of the above

29   Which of the following situations indicates the need for a reduced heparin dose on dialysis?

    A   When the patient has had a tooth extraction or oral surgery

    B   When the patient complains of dark, tarry stools

    C   Revision of the access post-dialysis

    D   Patient bleeds excessively post-dialysis

    E   All of the above

30   A variety of techniques are available and used to **prevent** the spread of infection. Of the following techniques listed, which one does **NOT** apply?

    A   Not eating or drinking in a dialysis unit

    B   Wearing Scrub suits

    C   Wearing Face shields

    D   Wearing of disposable gloves

    E   Putting on lip balm inside a dialysis unit is okay

31   Barrier precautions for infection control means:

    A   Isolating all HBV positive patients

    B   Isolating all HIV positive patients

    C   Vigorous hand-washing

    D   Wearing a face shield and gloves

    E   Wearing of protective clothing for body, face and hands

The following questions are either true or false. On the answer form, circle "T" for true and "F" for false.

32   T F   Methemoglobinemia is a condition where the hemoglobin portion of the RBC is unable to carry oxygen, causing the patient to exhibit fatigue and cyanosis.

33   T F   One parameter in assessing the uremic patient's state of nutrition is to evaluate their serum albumin. The acceptable range for the serum albumin is between 3.5 - 5.0 g/dL.

34   T F   Bleeding problems in dialysis patients may be related to a decrease in platelet adhesiveness.

35   T F   The heparin prescription is ideally based on the patient's body weight in kilograms and/or the clotting time studies.

36   T F   During hemodialysis, blood contacts foreign surfaces in the extracorporeal circuit requiring the use of an anticoagulant to prevent clotting.

37   T F   Alternative methods of assessing clotting of the extracorporeal circuit, in lieu of performing ACT's, include: frequent rinsing of the dialyzer with normal saline, observation of the drip chambers and dialyzers for clot and fibrin formation, and an increase in venous pressure during dialysis.

38   T F   In severe uremia, platelets have a tendency to lose their adhesiveness.

39   T F   An excessively low hematocrit may contribute to hypotension during dialysis.

40   T F   The term hemostasis means the checking or arrest (to stop) of blood flow from an injured blood vessel.

41   T F   The anemia of uremia is directly related to the decrease in the production of the hormone erythropoietin.

42   T F   Heparin Sodium USP has a *variable* molecular weight, ranging between 5,000 - 30,000 daltons and does not dialyze.

43   T F   Recombinant human erythropoietin has the same biological effects as endogenous erythropoietin.

44   T F   The term anticoagulation means against clotting.

45   T F   Prior to the initiation of recombinant human erythropoietin therapy, a patient's blood pressure should be adequately controlled.

46   T F   During dialysis, platelets have a tendency to increase their adhesiveness.

47   T F   Heparin Sodium USP is the drug of choice for dialysis to accomplish anticoagulation therapy. It is easy to administer and inhibits blood clotting by affecting all three stages of the clotting mechanism.

48   T F   Variables to consider with heparin requirements include: length of treatment, dialyzer membrane, blood flow rate and patient status (bleeding problems, high risk for bleeding, etc.).

49   T F   The differential count can be clinically significant in determining a patient's condition. It shows the average number of the different types of white blood cells and the typical normal percent for each respectively.

50   T F   The clotting complex in the blood is very complicated and occurs in a series of three stages.

51   T F   Tissue hypoxia stimulates erythropoiesis.

52   T F   A test dose of Iron Dextran Injection is recommended prior to intravenous administration of the drug to rule out anaphylactic and/or hypersensitivity reactions.

53   T F   Management of blood pressure is essential prior to initiation of recombinant human erythropoietin therapy. A simple method of accurately monitoring and tracking the patient's blood pressure is by calculating and tracking the mean arterial pressure.

54   T F   A complete blood count (CBC) can be obtained anytime during dialysis without affecting accurate test results.

55   T F   Plasma that is yellow in color, indicates hemolysis.

56   T F   In patient management during recombinant human erythropoietin therapy, folate and vitamin B_{12} deficiencies are carefully monitored.

57   T F   A low (1 - 2%) corrected reticulocyte count points to low bone marrow RBC output and hypoproliferative anemia, such as seen in ESRD.

58   T F   Avoid stopping the blood pump during dialysis, as stagnated blood will clot.

59   T F   Continuous heparinization during hemodialysis is preferred to the intermittent method to avoid clotting of the blood circuit.

60   T F   Using the recommended amount of normal saline and good priming technique, to remove all air from blood lines and dialyzer prior to patient use, will reduce the risk of extracorporeal clotting during dialysis.

Index